first place 4health

Bible Study Series

a joy-full season

Published by First Place 4 Health
Houston, Texas, U.S.A.
www.firstplace4health.com
Printed in the U.S.A.

© 2016 First Place 4 Health. All rights reserved.
978-1-942425-21-2

Unless otherwise indicated, Scripture quotations are taken from the *Holy Bible, New International Version*®. Copyright © 1973, 1978, 1984 by International Bible Society. Used by permission of Zondervan Publishing House. All rights reserved.

Other versions used include:

ESV—Scripture taken from the *English Standard Version*, Copyright © 2001. The *ESV* and *English Standard Version* are trademarks of Good News Publishers.

MSG—Scripture taken from *THE MESSAGE*. Copyright © by Eugene H. Peterson 1993, 1994, 1995, 1996, 2000, 2001, 2002. Used by permission of NavPress Publishing Group.

NKJV—Scripture taken from the *New King James Version*. Copyright © 1979, 1980, 1982 by Thomas Nelson, Inc. Used by permission. All rights reserved.

NLT—Scripture quotations marked *NLT* are taken from the *Holy Bible, New Living Translation*, copyright © 1996, 2004, 2007 by Tyndale House Foundation. Used by permission of Tyndale House Publishers, Inc., Carol Stream, Illinois 60188. All rights reserved.

Caution: The information contained in this book is intended to be solely informational and educational. It is assumed that the First Place 4 Health participant will consult a medical or health professional before beginning this or any other weight-loss or physical-fitness program.

contents

Introduction 5

Weekly Devotional Readings
Week One: We Give Thanks 9
Week Two: Our Answers to Prayer 27
Week Three: To Us a Son Is Given 47
Week Four: Do Not Be Afraid 67
Week Five: A New Creation 87
Week Six: Making a New Way 107

Additional Materials
Survival Tips 127
Leader Discussion Guide 135
First Place 4 Health Holiday Menus and Recipes 143
First Place 4 Health Member Survey 161
Personal Weight and Measurement Record 163
Weekly Prayer Partner Forms 165
Live It Trackers 177

introduction

*But seek first his kingdom and his righteousness,
and all these things will be given to you as well.*
MATTHEW 6:33

This book is not the typical First Place 4 Health Bible study. Instead, it is a special devotional tool to help you stay on course through the holidays, when many temptations will come your way. The Thanksgiving and Christmas holidays can be very busy with many social events, shopping expeditions, and church activities that make it difficult to remain faithful to your commitment to living healthy. This study was written to provide order in the hectic holiday season without being a burden on your time. It will give you inspiration for each day and also challenge you to stay on course by daily applying the truths at the core of First Place 4 Health.

One Scripture verse is featured each week, and the daily devotionals use that verse as the reference. The devotionals are holiday-related and give insight and encouragement to help you maintain balance during the holidays. A prayer and a journaling suggestion follow each reading. A journal page has also been provided for each day to write out your prayers, thoughts, and questions.

Holiday Survival Tips and menus for Thanksgiving, Christmas, and New Year's Day follow the six weeks of devotional readings. Holiday Survival Tips are valuable suggestions for helping you stay healthy spiritually, mentally, emotionally, and physically throughout the holiday season. Recipes for additional holiday favorites are included with the menus.

Also included at the back of *A Joy-Full Season* are weekly Prayer Partner forms and Live It Trackers. Fill out the weekly Prayer Partner form and put it into a basket during the meeting. After the meeting, you will draw out a prayer request form, and this will be your prayer partner for the week. The Live It Tracker is for you to complete at home and turn in to your leader at your weekly meeting.

If you have a plan, you can remain consistent in practicing the spiritual, mental, emotional, and physical disciplines you have begun in First Place 4 Health—even through the holidays!

My goals for this holiday season are:

Spiritual:

Mental:

Emotional: _____

Physical: _____

My strategies for reaching those goals are:

Spiritual: _____

Mental: _____

_____
_____
_____
_____
_____
_____

Emotional: _____

_____
_____
_____
_____
_____
_____

Physical: _____

_____
_____
_____
_____
_____
_____
_____

May the next six weeks take you on a joyful journey toward complete wholeness and health! Here's to the journey.

Week One

we give thanks

SCRIPTURE MEMORY VERSE
Now, our God, we give you thanks, and praise your glorious name.
1 CHRONICLES 29:13

WHEN YOU DON'T FEEL THANKFUL
by Lucinda Secrest McDowell

Day 1

Perhaps you aren't feeling thankful today. The world is a scary place. The losses have piled up one after another—health, relationships, financial security, dreams—and you really wish everyone would just quit asking you to list your one thousand gifts. . . . Some people call this *Turkey Day,* but that would be limiting. It is called *Thanksgiving* to prompt us to dig deep enough to find something that offers hope and promise. When I am in these hard places, I find it helpful to focus my soul on two things.

First, I remember that *God* is the One we thank. G.K. Chesterton once famously wrote, "The worst moment for an atheist is when he is really thankful and has no one to thank."[1] To whom are we thankful today? Our verse for the week reminds us that God is the One we praise. We thank Him because He loves us more than we can possibly imagine. He has our back. Knowing that we are created, loved, and sustained by a merciful and gracious God is the ultimate reason for giving thanks.

Second, I make a *choice* to live in gratitude, no matter what happens. I know I can either complain about the direction life has taken me—the detour in the road, the closed door, the seemingly impossible challenge—or I can believe *nothing is too hard for God-with-us* (that is, *Emmanuel*, one of the names of Jesus). Maybe your situation is darker this year than last, but if you know God as the Great Provider, you can choose to declare: "Though the fig tree does not bud and there are no grapes on the vines, though the olive crop fails and the fields produce no food, though there are no sheep in the pen and no cattle in the stalls, yet I will rejoice in the LORD, I will be joyful in God my Savior" (Habakkuk 3:17–18).

I'm grateful for parents who taught me early on that Thanksgiving is actually a way of life. Recently, I discovered a small piece of paper with a long childhood list—my "ticket" to Thanksgiving dinner. I was startled to count seventy different things on this thankful list—in categories, no less! If I could write that many at age twelve, just think of all I can thank God for today after so much more life and blessing.

What is *one thing* you can thank God for today? Even in the pain, even in the loneliness, even in the uncertainty? Now breathe it out or write it out. Good for you.

> *Heavenly Father, I thank You—most of all for loving me, for being my Savior and my Lord—but also for the many blessings You have showered on my life. Every good gift is from You, and I will declare my gratitude by living with a thankful heart. Not just on this holiday, but always. Amen.*

Journal: Write down something you can thank God for today that wasn't even on your radar last Thanksgiving. Now write someone who has touched your life in the past year for whom you are grateful.

I am thankful for our new Church + friends we have made there - for the blessing of my family being there for my Grandson & Daughter that was baptized —

I am thankful & blessed with my husband of 45 years, my kids and spouses Amber & Jason, my Grandkids that are so precious to me.

I miss my Mom & Dad and my brother but do know they are with our precious Father in heaven is my greatest blessing. I will see them again —

WHAT IF YOU DON'T FEEL LIKE THANKSGIVING?
by David Self

Day 2

One of my more forgettable Thanksgivings occurred when I was just turning thirteen. My dad was a minister, and we enjoyed a pretty modest life. I don't remember going to a lot of restaurants or eating fancy meals, but I do remember looking forward to Thanksgiving, when my mom and grandmother went all out in the kitchen. Few creatures enjoy consuming food like a growing teenage boy!

However, a few days before that Thanksgiving, dropping like dominoes, the entire Self clan developed a stomach virus. The last thing that we wanted on Thanksgiving Day was food! I thought that Thanksgiving was totally disappointing and totally forgettable. Yet as I matured in my years and in the faith, I learned that giving thanks often means we have to rise above circumstances. We must accept disappointments as a function of trying. Nothing ventured-nothing gained (and no room to be disappointed).

My lesson the Thanksgiving of my thirteenth year was that giving thanks to God and celebrating a national holiday must be about more than food and circumstances. There are so many reasons to be thankful. That lesson came back to me when I enrolled in First Place 4 Health. The first couple of weeks, try as I might, the scale wouldn't budge off my beginning weight. I tried to put a good face on the weight (pretend the number is your IQ), but the disappointment was real. Rather than giving thanks, I was bummed, discouraged, and wanted to quit.

Then I took the emphasis away from the food and began to thank God for His blessings: life, health, my church, my First Place 4 Health class and instructors, the ability to exercise, and a plan going forward. As the weeks passed, I rose above disappointment and followed the plan. As a result, the scale began to move in the right direction, and I had one more reason to give thanks.

Disappointment occurs when reality doesn't measure up to our expectations. If disappointment is left unchecked by God's Word and power, it can lead to doubt, defeat, discouragement, despair, and even depression. However, if, by faith, we focus on God and His blessings rather than disappointments, we can, in the words of the apostle Paul, "Give thanks in all circumstances; for this is God's will for you in Christ Jesus" (1 Thessalonians 5:18).

Dear Lord, today I choose to thank You for what You've given me. Help me not to focus on disappointments. Empower me to learn from setbacks, rise above discouragement, and do the next right thing. Amen.

Journal: Identify one disappointment that has turned into discouragement. Find at least one Scripture that helps point you back onto the road of thanksgiving.

Day 3: BEING A GOOD STEWARD
by Arla Frigstad

There I was, leading First Place 4 Health with a portable oxygen tank. The tank and I were inseparable for a month as I recovered from pneumonia and pulmonary embolisms. I tired easily and walked less than 500 steps a day. Before this happened, I was regularly walking more than twenty miles a week. The situation was serious, but I was thankful it was temporary and that I was able to recover quickly, according to my doctors, because I was in good shape. However, most of my life that had not been the case.

Because of First Place 4 Health, I became a regular exerciser about a year after I joined. I was at retirement age, yet I had never done strength training, regular exercise, or played competitive sports. Break a sweat? Never experienced it! Biceps, triceps, hip flexors . . . I knew I had them, but I had no idea where.

My inspiration has been my godson and my daughter-in-law. My godson died of ALS after an eight-year battle, leaving two young children. My daughter-in-law struggles daily with a neuromuscular disease that has taken away her mobility and her ability to do many things. It will continue to get worse unless a cure is found. Both of them would have dearly loved to play baseball, basketball, or other sports with their children, or simply take a walk, but they couldn't. They inspire me—and I want to be a good steward of the body God has given me.

What a waste it is for those of us who have the ability to exercise but do not. A close friend of a class member in my group is a mom with a disabled child. But the mom and child seldom go anywhere because the mom is obese, out of shape, and unable to lift her child's wheelchair or walk very far. So my friend, who has now lost about forty pounds, helps her.

That used to be my story. I am so thankful for this program that has helped me to appreciate what I have and provide a better home for the Holy Spirit within me. I can honor God by the choices I make—and because I weight-lift, I am strong enough to lift my daughter-in-law's electric scooter into the back of our van to take her shopping and on errands. A few years ago, I might not have been able. Are there opportunities in your life that you are missing because you are not in physical shape to help?

Father, You have given me this body. Help me to take better care of it. Help me push through when I don't feel like exercising. Help me to honor You with my body. Amen.

Journal: Are you giving God thanks for all that He has given you? Are your daily choices reflecting that thankfulness? Can you think of opportunities you might have missed, or might be in your future, for which you need to be in good physical shape? Write about this below.

Day 4

IS THERE ENOUGH?
by Beverly LaHote Schwind

The Bread of Life Rescue Mission is a place for the homeless and those who need a meal. It provides opportunities for the residents to find work, get on their feet, and learn about Jesus. The rules are strict, and all who stay there must attend the evening worship service.

My husband and I and five other couples take a meal to the mission once a month. This November marked the eighth year we have been doing this. We have seen the mission grow from a small kitchen in a house with four bedrooms and a church building that housed men in the basement (and sometimes cots upstairs), to a debt-free facility that can house fifty men on one side and fifty women on the other, plus a beautiful industrial kitchen and dining room.

Thanksgiving was a special time to serve in the new building. We talked about the menu we would present and how we could make it special. We served weeks before the holiday, but the entire month was a celebration of being in a new building. The founder of this mission was once in jail himself, and it was there he became a friend of Jesus and turned his life around. He had a vision to build a facility to help people get a new start. His church service is amazing, with people eager to give thanks to God and praise and honor His name.

November is usually a cold month here in Tennessee, so there are more people to feed. Recently, we were serving a large group that seemed to grow every time I looked up from the serving counter—lines of men, women, and children. We piled the food on their plates, eyeing the portions we had in our casseroles to the number of people. Usually we have an abundance of food and fewer people, so they come back for seconds and sometimes thirds. This night was different. We had enough for all the people who stayed at the mission, and the people who came off the street for a warm meal, but not many seconds.

They thanked us as they came through and picked up their warm meal. Then something happened that had never taken place before. A young woman came back and shyly asked for a second helping. I started to give it to her, and she said, "I'm sorry, have you eaten yet? Is there enough for you?" All of us in the serving line stopped and looked at her. No one had ever asked us if we had eaten. "We have that covered," I said. "This is for you." I smiled and scooped up some chicken pot pie on her plate, thankful there was some left.

Father God, we praise and thank You for the opportunity to serve. We are thankful that a day of thanks is every day. Help us to think of others and their needs—and not just at the holiday season. Amen.

Journal: Write about a time when you said you did not want something that was being served because you knew there would not be enough to go around. Or write about a time—maybe when you were a child—when someone did this for you so you could have a portion.

Day 5 — ATTITUDE OF GRATITUDE
by Judy Marshall

Each morning during my quiet time with God, I fill my heart, mind, and mouth with praise to the Lord. I marvel at His creation and creativity, His love and generosity, His power and might. Then, closing my Bible, I walk away from my quiet place into the "dailyness" of life. I fail to carry my worship with me as I begin the daily physical walk of First Place 4 Health.

Reluctantly, I meet my morning exercise group. My feet are heavy and do not want to walk those three miles today. I become overwhelmed with the time and effort it takes to plan and prepare healthy meals, and I just shrug at my Tracker. Most always, I meet temptations, either with my hands hanging limp at my side or tied behind my back.

How can the five minutes between worship with God and my first choice take such a downward turn? What happened to praising God? Can you relate to this kind of day? Resenting exercise turns aside God's joy of knitting my form into His own. Fretting over meal preparation and tracking takes away my enjoyment of cooking and eating healthy food. Falling prey to every temptation allows my enemy to devour any chance of victory. All this comes quickly on the heels of praise and thanksgiving!

Is there hope? Of course. After all, I am His child! I just have to realize my entire day is really His and for His glory. Closing my Bible in the morning does not end my worship; it is to continue all day long. So now, when dailyness begins to invade God's worship and praise, I will quickly press pause and turn my complaining into gratitude.

Exercise . . . instead of "ugh!" I will say, "Thank You, Lord, for creating my body to move with balance and grace. Thank You for the time and ability to walk and Your faithfulness to meet me on my first step. Thank You for friends who walk beside me."

Meal planning and preparation . . . instead of "oh, dear!" I will say, "Thank You, Lord, for the gift of food and Your generous provision. I praise You for creating so many healthy varieties that are readily available. Thank You for the opportunity to make healthy choices and to meet my family's physical needs."

Temptations . . . instead of saying nothing, I will raise my hands and say, "Lord, I praise Your glorious name! I need Your power to turn away from this and to make the healthy choice You have placed before me. Your victory allows my victory, and I thank You!"

Keeping an attitude of gratitude is essential in First Place 4 Health. It is impossible to separate worship, thanksgiving, and praise. A grateful heart is praise and worship to God . . . all day long! And as we continually worship Him, we are continually in His presence.

God, thank You for being our God and for being available to hear our grateful hearts offer praise to Your glorious name. Help us to quickly turn our ungrateful attitude to gratitude for all You are—for You are all we desire. Amen.

Journal: Make a list of three complaints in your life today. In each one, find two reasons to give thanks and praise to God. This will become your act of worship.

THE SOUND OF MUSIC
by Pat Lewis

Day 6

Our family gathers at my home each year for Thanksgiving, and we normally share the things for which we are thankful before our meal. Last year we had late-comers, and everyone was anxiously awaiting the meal. As they finally arrived and began to move toward the food, I said, "Wait! I have some things I want to tell you that I'm thankful for this year." My guests, thinking this was time for all to share, moaned and sat down. Then I began to read a list of cleanup chores that I was thankful for when they cheerfully helped me. We all had a good laugh as we gathered around the food and gave thanks to our Father for His bountiful provision.

I love to give thanks and praise to our Lord and Savior Jesus Christ. I sing praise and thanksgiving to Him in my quiet time. I have an older voice now that crackles, but He doesn't seem to mind. Psalm 100:4 says to "come before Him with joyful song," and Psalm 105:2 says "sing to Him, sing praise to Him." The more time I spend with Him, the more I just want to thank Him for who He is and for all His wondrous works.

Music stirs my heart as nothing else, and I have always loved singing. In fact, the old hymn *Almost Persuaded*, sung in a church revival as a young person, influenced my salvation. Being a lover of hymns and some of the new praise songs, I have searched the Internet, old hymnals, and other sources in the last few years for songs to add to my daily journal. In one of the old hymnals I found this declaration by Martin Luther—who wrote hymns that also influenced singing in the churches:

> *I wish to see all arts, principally music, in the service of Him who gave and created them. Music is a fair and glorious gift of God. I would not for the world forgo my humble share of music. Singers are never sorrowful, but are merry, and smile through their troubles in song. Music makes people kinder, gentler, more staid and reasonable. I am strongly persuaded that after theology there is no art than can be placed on the level with music; for beside theology, music is the only art capable of affording peace and joy of the*

heart . . . the devil flees before the sound of music almost as much as before the Word of God.

First Place 4 Health encourages members to have a quiet time each day to give thanks and praise to our Lord and Savior through praying God's Word, reading Scriptures, Bible study, and other methods of choice. You may want to add a song of praise to your daily time with Him. As we learn from Martin Luther, He is the One "who gave and created them."

Our Father, creator of heaven and earth and song, I enter Your gates with thanksgiving and Your courts with praise. I will give thanks to You and praise Your name, for You, Lord, are good and Your love endures forever. Amen.

> **Journal:** Jesus said to go into a closet and close the door when we pray (see Matthew 6:6). Find a quiet place in your home or out in nature to give thanks, praise, and worship to our glorious God. Journal your favorite hymn or praise song.

AT THE FEET OF JESUS
by Sherry Leggett

Day 7

When the holidays roll around, my to-do list starts out with an unchecked box labeled "Be Everything to Everyone," which clearly demonstrates my Type E personality. By the time the holidays actually begin, my to-do list is so overwhelming that my hands get clammy, my heart starts pounding, my breath quickens, and I take an oath I'm getting a cold. It's so easy for a to-do list to snowball out of control. In some cases, it takes no time at all to go from "I can do this" to outright panic. It reminds me of someone in the Bible who also had a Type E personality.

Jesus and His disciples went to Mary and Martha's house for dinner. I'm sure Martha was the "hostess with the mostest." She probably was gifted in making people feel at home. In my mind, her house could have been displayed in Jerusalem's *Better Homes and Gardens* magazine. But while Martha was running around doing a to-do list that probably rivaled mine this morning, her sister was sitting at the feet of Jesus.

In the heat of the moment, when Martha was experiencing her to-do list panic, she called out Mary and said to Jesus, "Tell her to lend me a hand." Jesus replied, "Martha, dear Martha, you're fussing far too much and getting yourself worked up over nothing. One thing only is essential, and Mary has chosen it" (Luke 10:40–42, *MSG*).

Let that sink into your Type E soul: *one thing only is essential.* In 1 Thessalonians 5:16–18, Paul states, "Rejoice always, pray continually, give thanks in all circumstances." The cure for the Type E personality—being everything to everyone—is to pray continually at the feet of Jesus and give thanks in all circumstances. We were created to have an attitude of gratitude. In fact, research studies show that grateful people have healthier habits (such as exercising), a healthier diet, and better stress management. Being grateful can even boost our immune system so we don't get that cold.

The cure for Type E personality isn't doing more. It's the opposite . . . just stopping, listening for God, and looking at His world for the little things He creates to teach us. For me, my heart rate returns to normal when I sit at the feet of Jesus, give thanks to Him, and purposefully write in my gratitude journal. "Now, our God, we give You thanks, and praise Your glorious name."

Dear Lord, thank You for putting my busyness into perspective when I sit at Your feet. I was created to do one thing—to praise You and Your glorious name. Amen.

Journal: Start your own gratitude journal by writing three things that you are thankful for today. Try to maintain this journaling throughout the season.

Note
1. G.K. Chesterton, quoted in *St. Francis of Assisi* (1923).

Group Prayer Requests

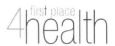

Today's Date: _____

Name	Request

Results

_____
_____
_____
_____
_____

Week Two

our answers to prayer

SCRIPTURE MEMORY VERSE
I will give you thanks, for you answered me; you have become my salvation.
PSALM 118:21

DAY 1: HE LISTENS
by Becky Turner

Day 1

When I was a little girl, I remember a missionary coming to speak to my class at Vacation Bible School. He enthralled us with stories of life on the mission field and how God "spoke" to him and led him to do certain things. His relationship with the Lord seemed so real and viable, and I left class that day asking God to speak to me. I wanted to hear His voice.

As an adult, I still desire to hear from the Lord. But something I have become more and more aware of is His desire to hear from me. In fact, every time I draw near to Him and lift my voice in prayer, petition, or thanksgiving, I can be confident that God inclines His ear to hear me. This makes my heart glad and gives me a confident trust in my relationship with Him.

Amazingly, I am in good company. Jesus Himself was thankful to know that His Father was always listening, and He let us know it just before He called Lazarus out from the tomb. "So they took away the stone. Then Jesus looked up and said, 'Father, I thank you that you have heard me. I knew that you always hear me'" (John 11:41–42).

Jesus knew that His Father always heard Him, and He said so for our benefit. As we gather around our bountiful tables this Thanksgiving and count our blessings one by one before our Father, may we rejoice to know that He hears us. And let us not only give thanks for Him to hear but also that others may know the things He has done for us and the things we are expecting in the days to come!

First John 5:14–15 is one of my favorite Scriptures concerning prayer. It says, "This is the confidence we have in approaching God: that if we ask anything according to his will, he hears us. And if we know that he hears us—whatever we ask—we know that we have what we asked of him." For me, the greatest part of this Scripture is not the knowing that we can have what we ask but the revelation that God hears us when we call out to Him.

God hears our thankful hearts. He hears our cries in the night. He hears us when we are in need and petition Him. He hears us when we cry out in weakness and vulnerability. He hears us in times of temptation when we need His strength to overcome. God is faithful, and just as much as we desire to hear from Him, He desires to hear from us.

Lord God, thank You that You hear us when we call out to You.
Thank You that Your throne room is always open to us and that we may
come in and tell You what is pressing on our heart. Thank You that You hear
the prayers we lift up throughout the day. Amen.

Journal: List something that has become a worry or concern to you this week. Write out your need before the Lord and know that, whether written or spoken, He hears you and has your answer today!

our answers to prayer

Day 2 DO THE NEXT RIGHT THING
by Carole Lewis

Yesterday was the fourteenth anniversary of the death of our daughter, Shari, in 2001. She was hit by an eighteen-year-old girl who was driving drunk on Thanksgiving night as her family prepared to leave her in-law's home. She left behind her husband, Jeff, and three daughters, who were thirteen, fifteen, and nineteen at the time.

I felt I was dealing with the anniversary okay, but when I awoke this morning I realized that my eating had been out of control for the last week. God was gracious to show me that it had been triggered by giving in to the feelings of helplessness to change history. As I prayed and thanked God for taking care of all of us these past fourteen years, I realized that once again I had failed to trust Him with my own life and the lives of those I love.

So what do I do right here, right now? I got up this morning and took my own advice to "do the next right thing." I made a pot of steel-cut oatmeal, full of apples, raisins, Craisins, cinnamon, and vanilla. I made a bowl of tuna salad and Mason jar salads to eat this week leading up to Thanksgiving. God is always faithful to show us what is going on, if we will only stop and ask Him. After we become aware of what we are doing and why we are doing it, we always have the opportunity to stop the destructive behavior and go back in the right direction.

It distresses me that after losing thirty pounds over the course of the last two years, I am just a binge away from going back to my old ways. Success continues to be a three-part plan:

1. God will give me the strength
2. Others will encourage me
3. I am the only one who can do the hard work of change

I know myself well, and because the Holy Spirit lives inside of me, He showed me the way back—once again. I must accept that Thanksgiving is only one day, and overeating one day will not cause weight gain. It is overeating leading up to the holiday . . . and then continuing to overeat during the holidays until the dawn of the New Year.

Many of us have emotional pain associated with past holidays, and our way of dealing with that pain is to stuff it down with food. God wants to heal our heart and set us on a new path, but there are three things we must do to move forward: (1) acknowledge our pain; (2) ask for God's help to change; and (3) do the next right thing. As we repeat these steps each time the pain resurfaces, slowly and surely God will heal our broken hearts.

Lord God, thank You for hearing our pleas for strength when we are weak and tempted to make poor choices for our body, mind, or spirit. Thank You for showing us when we are making bad choices and for helping us get back on track. Thank You that when we call, You answer us. Amen.

Journal: Think about some of the sources of stress that you are anticipating for the upcoming holiday season. Write out your concerns to God and ask Him to give you the strength, wisdom, and perseverance to "do the next right thing."

Day 3 — WAIT AND PRAY
by Helen Baratta

"Why so long, Lord?" My toes tap, my knee jiggles, and my thoughts race whenever I wait. The time passes ever so slowly. If I had known in my wellness journey that it would take me four years to lose 116 pounds and reach a healthy weight, I would have never started. I would have thought the wait too long, too hard, and too impossible.

Yet the long length of time it has taken me to lose weight has helped me adjust to the different lifestyle I needed to navigate the difficulties of maintenance. I am thankful for the time I've spent asking for God's help. Slowly, I walked from the chains of obesity to freedom.

God hears our prayers. As He promises in His Word, "Call to me and I will answer you and tell you great and unsearchable things you do not know" (Jeremiah 33:3). Are you praying for a breakthrough? Have you asked God for victory? Are you weary of waiting for an answer? Then strengthen your faith as you wait and PRAY:

> **P**ay attention: You can't hear the answer to your prayers when you allow worries, fears, and busyness to dictate your life. Distractions are like the thorns in Luke 8:7 that "grew up with [the seed] and choked the plants." Eliminate the thorns and pay attention to God at work in your life.
>
> **R**each for God: "But seek first his kingdom and his righteousness, and all these things will be given to you as well" (Matthew 6:33). Just as children gain comfort and security when they stretch to grab the hand of a parent, our relationship with our heavenly Father deepens as we reach out to Him. Spend time reading and studying the Bible. Allow God's Word to penetrate your heart.
>
> **A**cknowledge God as Lord: "Trust in the LORD with all your heart, and lean not on your own understanding; in all your ways acknowledge Him, and he shall direct your paths" (Proverbs 3:5–6 NKJV). When you recognize God as Lord of your life, you acknowledge the authority He has in your life. You will experience His peace as you relinquish control.
>
> **Y**earn to know more about God: "If any of you lacks wisdom, you should ask God, who gives generously to all without finding fault, and it will be given to you" (James 1:5). May we never cease yearning to know more of God.

Lord, thank You for Your abounding love. Show me the distractions in my life that crowd out Your voice. I want to choose what is best, so help me prioritize my time with You. Give me wisdom as I yearn to know You more. You are Almighty God, and I will wait for You. My salvation is in You. Amen.

Journal: Write out and pray Psalm 27, substituting your name in each verse.

JOY TO MY HEART
by Barb Lukies

Day 4

This week's verse reminds me of when I began my journey in 2002. I was obese and desperately needed to lose weight, but I wanted help spiritually as well. I prayed and asked God to provide a Christian mentor who could support me in my journey. Little did I know that God had it all planned with the perfect answer—First Place 4 Health, a Christian total health program that provided educational resources in fitness, nutrition, and health as well as Bible study, prayer support, and encouragement from a small-group setting. This put the focus on God and helped me change mentally, physically, spiritually, and emotionally.

As I was clearing out some cupboards recently, I came across a stack of cards I had saved from previous members and leaders I had met during First Place 4 Health. It brought so much joy to my heart, and I was so thankful for each and every word on the notes. God spoke into my life not just when I first received them but also years later when I read them again. Some of the cards were notes of encouragement to keep going in my journey toward a healthier life in Christ. One note in particular caught my eye: "Because of your prayers, I became a Christian, and I wanted to thank you for putting the salvation prayer on the online group boards." There is such great joy in seeing others give their lives to Christ through this program.

There has been many times over the years when I have prayed for members and their families. God answered each and every prayer in His timeframe and in accordance to His will for their lives. I still give thanks daily for all He has done and continues to do in and through their lives. I often look back over my past prayer journals and write thank-you notes to God in my thankfulness journals for the answered prayers.

I give thanks for each person who has enriched my life and pointed me back to a real and lasting relationship with Christ. Today, God has continued to work through people in the First Place 4 Health program, even years after meeting them for the first time. From time to time, I get Facebook, SMS messages, and emails sent to me from members across the world asking for prayer. It is a privilege to pray with them and see God answer their prayers.

Lord, I pray that I will look for ways to encourage others in my daily life. Open my heart to those who need encouragement. Amen.

Journal: This holiday season, reflect back on whom God has placed in your life to support you spiritually, mentally, emotionally, and physically. List some of your prayers that God has answered.

Day 5 — I WILL GIVE YOU THANKS
by Wendy Lawton

The table was set. The turkey, trimmed with root vegetables and stuffed with savory dressing, took center stage. All the family favorites were lined up: candied yams, corn pudding, creamed onions, mashed potatoes, rich gravy, Grandma's yeast rolls, green bean casserole, cranberry sauce, olives . . . the table fairly groaned under the feast. The fragrance of the food set everyone's stomachs to growling. But before they began, there was one tradition. From the oldest to the youngest, each person seated at the table had to say for what they were thankful.

Grandfather started out. Looking around the table, he said that he was thankful for his family and another year to enjoy them. Grandma was next, then Mom and Dad, and then onto the children. Jason said he was thankful for food and football and that they were almost done with telling their thanks. Jen, being the youngest at eleven, was next. She said she was thankful for Thanksgiving. Dad smiled and asked her if she knew why we celebrate. Jason kicked her under the table and mouthed, "Hurry up. I'm hungry."

Jen knew the answer. They'd studied it in school during the last week. "The Pilgrims first celebrated Thanksgiving, and we do it to remember them."

Dad had one more question. "So, Jen, who were they thanking?"

"That's easy, Dad. It was in my textbook. They invited the Indians to thank them for saving them from starving during their first winter."

Dad was quiet for a moment. "Let's discuss this more as we eat," he said. "Grandpa, will you ask a blessing on this food?"

So, what was wrong with Jen's answer? She was right that we remember the Pilgrims on Thanksgiving. But she was wrong that they were thanking the Indians—the Native Americans who welcomed them to their land and helped them through that awful first winter. The Pilgrims invited their native neighbors to join them in thanking *God* for seeing them through. Too many families sit around their Thanksgiving table and recount the things for which they are grateful, completely forgetting to offer thanks to the One who provided all that they mentioned.

This week's verse is one the Pilgrims knew well. They offered up their thanks to the One who answered their prayers—to the One who saved them. They invited their new friends to join them in thanking God. This Thanksgiving, as we are gathered around the table, let us also encourage each family member and guest to direct their thanks to the One who has answered us and saved us.

Father, we learn great lessons from those witnesses who have gone before us, like the Pilgrims. Let us stop and give You thanks for provision and for our own salvation. Amen.

Journal: Don't be afraid to list the things for which you are grateful this year. But this time, write it as a thank-you note to God.

Day 6: ANSWERED PRAYERS
by Megan Heath Keefe

Have you ever thought about how important an answer can be? In this week's verse, the psalmist is saying that answers are something for which we should be thankful—whether yes, no, or maybe—and whether the answers are what we were expecting or not. Now *that* is a healthy attitude of the heart.

When we were children, we heard the answer "no" a lot. As teenagers, we probably heard quite a few "maybes." Now as adults, we should be hearing a lot of "yes's," because we are mature enough to know for what to ask. Any of these answers can bring peace, comfort, anticipation, security, and even sadness.

As I have grown in my relationship with Jesus Christ, I have come to the place where I am genuinely grateful for any answers from Him. I have discovered that the more time I spend with Jesus, the better I am at hearing and accepting His answers to my prayers. These answers have literally been my salvation at times.

I prayed for years for a godly husband. The answer was a definite yes, but I had to be patient for God to reveal him. I prayed for children, and the Lord said, "No, not yet; there will be time soon for a baby." Now I have a two-year old and one on the way!

As I reflect this Thanksgiving, it does my heart good to remember all the answered prayers. I have to admit that the happiest memories I have are the ones I remember when God said "yes." But I have to wonder how grateful I would have been if the answer had been "no" or "not now."

I am praying for a deeper acceptance of God's will for my life in all things. I am praying for a real understanding that His answers are sometimes for my protection, for my wellbeing, and for His glory. If God would have said yes to everything I asked Him for in the past ten years, I would not have my precious godly husband or my children. Most of all, I would have missed His best for me.

What are the answers you are looking for this Thanksgiving season? God's timing is always perfect.

Lord, as I lend my ear to Your voice, teach me to trust You, regardless of the answer. Amen.

Journal: Reflect on the answered prayers of this past year and give thanks for them. Be faithful to continue to listen for those answers that are yet to come.

DAILY THANKFULNESS
by Karen Porter

Day 7

At the close of a First Place 4 Health class, each member completed this sentence: "Today, I am thankful for _____." One by one the sentence was finished with grateful words, thanking God for husbands, wives, children, opportunities, health, and freedom. One member said, "I'm thankful the Lord hears me."

The psalmist who wrote this week's verse thanked God for hearing and answering. We don't often praise God because He hears us. We seem to expect His attention. And often when He responds we aren't grateful—especially for the small answers.

What if we began to thank and praise God in quick short prayers of gratitude instead of waiting to say a long formal prayer? The psalmist thanked God for hearing. We can thank God for small blessings too. For friends who care. A warm home. A good night's sleep. A sweet conversation with a ten-year-old. Rearranged furniture in a well-lived room. Healthy food. A place to walk. A pound lost. A clear blue sky after a storm.

If we thank God daily (and hourly) for small treasures, we will begin to see how He is engaged in all our activities. He cares for us. He orders our steps. He clears the path before us. He sends beauty and joy our way. Thanking God for what seems obvious gives Him credit as the creator and sustainer of life and allows us to see the bigger picture of His mercy and protection and provision.

Ann Voskamp writes that it is possible to see and seek God in *everything*. "And if the eyes gaze long enough to see God lifted in a thing, how can the lips not offer *eucharisteo* [thanksgiving]."[1] It's true. If we open our eyes, God will be lifted up.

Paul said, "Always [give] thanks to God the Father for everything" (Ephesians 5:20 NLT). Thank Him for salvation through Jesus Christ. Thank Him for sunshine and rain. Thank Him for First Place 4 Health and the opportunity to get fit and healthy. Thank Him for flowers and moonlight. He is gracious to give you salvation and hope, and He is kind enough to wrap your life in beauty and joy. God loves quick thanksgiving. So don't delay your praise.

Lord, You are the God of gifts—big and small. Open my eyes to see You in every moment. Give me lips of praise. Amen.

Journal: List some of the small treasures for which you are thankful today.

Note

1. Ann Voskamp, *One Thousand Gifts* (Grand Rapids, MI: Zondervan, 2010), p. 114.

Group Prayer Requests

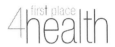

Today's Date: _____

Name	Request

Results

_____
_____
_____
_____
_____

Week Three

to us a son is given

Scripture Memory Verse

For to us a child is born, to us a son is given, and the government will be on his shoulders. And he will be called Wonderful Counselor, Mighty God, Everlasting Father, Prince of Peace.
Isaiah 9:6

DON'T MISS CHRISTMAS
by Vicki Heath

Day 1

Worry, hurry, traffic, presents, shopping, the tree, food, kids, money, food, family, party, food, and more food. And we are supposed to take time and celebrate the birth of Christ? My heart's desire is to focus on the incarnation, but all the busyness can be a distraction. God does not want the celebration of the birth of His Son to be anything but joyful. The craziness of Christmas does not have to consume us. We can experience the true meaning of Christmas in the midst of all of the family and functions of the season.

The secret of enjoying every moment of the Christmas season is found in Isaiah 9:6, this week's verse. Jesus is called *Wonderful Counselor*, and He is. He said in Matthew 6 not to worry about where the money for presents will come from, or Christmas clothes, or how to decorate our house. If He can take care of the birds in the air and the flowers of the field, He can surely take care of us. So let's not allow guilt or shame or television commercials to dictate how much we spend on our Christmas.

Instead, let's seek the guidance of our Wonderful Counselor and pray. He will lead us to the perfect, meaningful, and creative season of giving.

Jesus is also called the Prince of Peace—and nobody does peace like Jesus, for He Himself is our peace. God's peace can reign over our homes during the season if we seek the Prince. He will be our focus and how we start our day if we ask the Prince to come and reign supremely over our holiday season. We can ask Him to rain down His peace on us and our house. After all, it is His birthday.

Dear Father, help me to willingly cast my cares on Your strong shoulders. Remind me by Your Holy Spirit that You are there for me and that You are totally capable of carrying anything I throw Your way. Amen.

Journal: Write a few things today that you need to cast on the strong and mighty shoulders of our Messiah.

HIS NAME
by Karen Porter

Day 2

We searched through the lists and charts that contained our family records, finding names as far back as the 1700s. I loved how the names repeated themselves in later generations. A son was named William after a great grandfather, or a daughter was named Maddie after an aunt.

Then I noticed a name that popped up five or six times. Several girls were named *America*. After a bit of research, we discovered the first family that had arrived here was so grateful that they named their first daughter after the country they now loved. I wished I had known about the name before I named my children. When my daughter saw the history, she gave the name to her daughter.

Names matter. We choose names from our family repertoire established over generations. Some researchers even say names affect our destiny—noting there are a disproportionately large number of dentists named Dennis and lawyers named Lauren. One writer said it is no accident that the Greathouse family in West Virginia runs a real-estate firm. Bible names often have meanings beyond the moniker of the person named. Esther's name means *star*. Nehemiah's name means *comforted*. Theophilus means *friend of God*.

When Isaiah predicted the Savior would be born, he couldn't give the child only one name. He listed several. *Wonderful Counselor. Mighty God. Everlasting Father. Prince of Peace.* And Isaiah's list is short—there are hundreds more names for Christ in Scripture. Mary gave the baby the name *Jesus*, as the angel instructed: "And behold, you will conceive in your womb and bear a son, and you shall call his name Jesus. He will be great and will be called the Son of the Most High. And the Lord God will give to him the throne of his father David, and he will reign over the house of Jacob forever, and of his kingdom there will be no end" (Luke 1:31-33 ESV).

From Genesis to the end of the New Testament, the Bible paints a portrait of Jesus with names. In the four names listed in this Isaiah package, we see Him clearly. He is our *counselor*—we can tell Him anything and He will help us find solutions, answers, and clarity. He is our *God*—we can depend on Him for provision, protection, and power. He is our *Father*—we can be sure He always has our best interests in mind even when He tells us "no" or "wait." He is *Peace*—we have no need to struggle with worry and anxiety in life, because He sheds peace over every situation.

There is power in the wonderful names of our Lord—and power to be claimed by calling Him each one.

> *Jesus, Your names are powerful, meaningful, and life giving. I praise You for being our Great Light, our Sanctuary, and our King. Thank You for being our Refiner, our Source, and our Friend. Amen.*

Journal: List areas where you need the Lord's help in finding solutions and answers. Are you trusting Him with these answers, even if the answer is "wait"?

Day 3: HOLDING ON TO THE PROMISE
by Martha Rogers

God had a plan for His Son and for humankind from the beginning of time. God revealed that plan to Isaiah and many other prophets in the Old Testament. Each one of us has been a part of that plan. God gave us free will—the opportunity to make choices that affect our lives.

When you choose to be in a First Place 4 Health class, you make a choice to do what is best for your body, mind, spirit, and heart. You make choices every day. Some will impact only that day, but some will impact your future. Choosing to take care of your body through physical exercise and healthy eating is a choice that means you want to live a healthier life. Spending time with the Lord each morning in prayer and Bible study gives you a healthier spirit and a deeper relationship with the Lord.

You will face challenges, even as Jesus faced the challenges from the Pharisees and Sanhedrin. Jesus walked on this earth, and people had trouble accepting the truth He brought. Those who did found the peace that passes all understanding and entered into the purpose of it all. Through the birth and death of Jesus, and the Holy Spirit, you can now have a close relationship with God the Father and Jesus, His Son. When challenges come, you can remember that you have a Wonderful Counselor and a Prince of Peace who will guide you and walk with you every step of the way.

Through these Old Testament prophecies, God gave us His plan, His promise, and His purpose. In our First Place 4 Health experience, God gives us the health plan. He promises to walk with us, and His purpose is to draw us closer to Him. Whether we are trying to lose weight and be healthy or maintain what we have achieved, God is our Peace, our Everlasting Father, and our Almighty God. This week's verse holds a promise for everyone: it tells of a child to be born who will be the One with the government of the world on His shoulders. That child would be the Savior who would die to forgive our sins and redeem our lives.

As we celebrate Christmas this year, let us think about the plan, the prophecy, the promise, and the purpose that God gave us through His Son, Jesus Christ. When we remember these four things, His peace will reign in our hearts throughout turmoil and storms and joy and happiness. Jesus fulfilled the plan, through God's promise, and He is the Prince of Peace, the everlasting Father. He is the Light to scatter the darkness, and He is the Love that knows no end and has no conditions.

Heavenly Father, thank You for the gift of Your Son, Jesus Christ.
May we never forget the love You have for us even in our transgressions.
May this be a time of rejoicing for the Savior of the World. Amen.

Journal: Write down any challenges you have faced in the past year. Write a prayer thanking God for seeing you through these challenges. For those you are still facing, pray for His power and strength to fill you as you walk through each situation.

week three

NO PROBLEM
by Beverly LaHote Schwind

Day 4

Night after night I tossed and turned, wanting to tell my husband but somehow feeling that if I did, it wouldn't happen. A recent discussion with our friends on the expenses of a family haunted me. Jim had remarked, "Three children are enough!" All had agreed. My spirit sunk. *Three children are enough,* I thought. *But that isn't the way it's going to be.* I had to tell him soon. Would he resent this child? Would he blame me for being careless? Why was I taking all the blame? I would be the one with the extra work and fewer hours of sleep.

Unable to sleep one night, I wandered into the living room. I stared out of the picture window of our small suburban home. The trees were illuminated by the full moon, their branches looking thin and naked as they reached skyward and cast black shadows on the white ground. "Oh, God," I prayed, "help me cope with this. I'm not doing a very good job." I couldn't help remembering another prayer of mine ten years before when I was childless. Like Hannah in the Bible, I had prayed for a child. God had heard my prayer then. Was I ungrateful now?

As I stood deep in thought and prayer, a warm hand touched my shoulder. "What's bothering you, honey?" Jim asked. Suddenly, all the stored-up emotions surfaced. My sobs made it impossible to speak. He held me close until I was able to compose myself and mutter, "Jim, I'm pregnant." Silence . . . but it felt good just to say the words. He gently stroked my bangs, a gesture I usually hated but I now welcomed.

"No problem," he said, "we have enough love for another child." He had turned my fears into joy. I began to look expectantly for the coming of this new member of our family.

Mary, no doubt, knew of Isaiah's prophetic words that a Savior would be born, but I think when it became a reality to her, she had many thoughts and questions. She was concerned what her future husband would think. Her reassurance from visiting Elizabeth, who was with child, must have confirmed for her that the words of Isaiah were coming to pass.

The angels declared to the shepherds that the baby was born, and Scripture tells us it was good news and great joy. The joy was so great that after the angel announced it to the shepherds, the great company of heavenly host could not contain themselves. They all joined in praising, "Glory to God in the highest, and on earth peace, goodwill toward men" (Luke 2:14 NKJV). All of heaven rejoiced.

God's timing is always right. He brought us the exact daughter we needed in our lives. She has brought us great joy, plus five granddaughters and a great-grandson who are an active part of our lives. I am thankful that God sent Jesus into the world to be our Messiah.

Thank You, holy Christ Child, for coming into this world. As we celebrate Your birth, may we feel the excitement of the heavenly host as we praise You and sing the Christmas carols. Amen.

Journal: Write about a time when you were worried about something. How did you resolve the situation? How did it help to share your concern with others?

Day 5 PRINCE OF PEACE
by Wendy Lawton

Halloween is barely over when magazines and Pinterest boards fill with ideas for Christmas. Martha Stewart is cooking up a feast that cannot possibly be recreated without a staff of sous chefs. The recipes for cookies and cakes and pastries are endless.

In my first years of marriage, I bought *Good Housekeeping* and tried to replicate their Christmas décor, never realizing the budget for those rooms was more than we made in a year. My scaled-down efforts always ended up deeply disappointing. One year I went all out and made a two-story gingerbread house, complete with sugar-glazed windows and electric lighting. Unfortunately, I was so exhausted when I finished that I could hardly wrap gifts or cook a meal.

It took me years to realize those glossy magazine pages were my own brand of temptation. No, I did not need to bake seventeen different cookies for my family and friends. We did not need it. It was a subtle form of gluttony.

And gifts . . . I cringe each Christmas when the luxury car companies come out with ads showing their $80,000 cars wrapped with big red bows. *The perfect gift.* Or diamonds. Or expensive electronics. Talk about stress! In 2015, the average American spent $830 on gifts at Christmas. That's up fifteen percent from 2014.[1] And most of that goes on credit cards.

Creating meals for guests at Christmas holds the same dangers. Why do we think we have to stretch to gourmet standards and offer more food than anyone can possibly eat? At First Place 4 Health we're committed to eating healthy, right? So why don't we continue to cook healthy, simple, delicious meals at Christmas? Our guests will thank us for caring for their health as well as ours.

I still love to decorate, but we now have beloved ornaments and the same two trees, the same nativity, and the same table décor every year. Our children come home to their cherished memories instead of an expensive new "theme" each year. Over-scheduling and over-reaching is just as dangerous. In this week's verse, Isaiah foretells that the child who was to come would be the Prince of Peace. Christmas should be a season of peace, not a season of overdoing it to the point of stress.

Father, You are the Prince of Peace, and You long to bring peace into our lives. Help us stay focused on the lasting things at Christmastime—to use the season as a time to celebrate Your birth. Let it be a time of peace, not a time of stress. Amen.

Journal: Write down the things you want to do this Christmas. Now assign each a number: #1 are things that will deepen your faith or relationships; #2 are things that bring pleasure; #3 are chores that meet expectations; #4 are those things you dread. Look over your list. Can they all be done while making the season one of peace and fulfillment? If not, what can you cross off?

Day 6

TRUSTING GOD
by Sherry Leggett

Every day of the week, my job requires me to practically wear pillows on my feet—that is, my blissful running shoes. For special occasions, I have an adorable pair of black and white, super chic, towering, high heels. I love them, but they are my "church only" shoes. When I wear these trendy shoes, I can feel all twenty-six bones, thirty-three joints, 100 muscles, and all the tendons and ligaments in each foot.

Not only are they my "church only" shoes, but they are also my "church only *if* I'm not teaching Sunday School or making an announcement" shoes. When I arrive home from church, these shoes are off my tortured feet before I'm out of the car. I promptly put the aesthetically pleasing shoes on a high shelf in a box until the next time I decide to brave high fashion over staying comfortable. Like my trendy shoes, we often put on a smile for our First Place 4 Health group or church. We work hard so no one knows our grief or pain (like my feet and ankles).

Isaiah 9:6 shows all the glory that Jesus would be born into even though He was a child. People were waiting on a majestic event when Jesus was born humbly into a manager. The angels appeared to shepherds, a class of people who were not even permitted in the temple at that time. Even the birth of Jesus was littered with events that weren't considered royal in the eyes of the people.

This humble birth made Jesus the *Wonderful Counselor*—one to seek when things aren't going well in our lives. He will give us guidance. In my life, sometimes that guidance has come through my First Place 4 Health group and Bible studies. He also became the *Mighty God* and *Everlasting Father*, who is bigger than all our struggles on our journey to wellness in our mind, body, spirit, and emotions. And He became the *Prince of Peace,* who has no limits to the wholeness and comfort He can bring to our lives.

Jesus understands what it means to be broken in every sense of the word. We can't be healed our hurts, pains, or pasts by trying harder to live a good life and cover up our raggedness. But if we take off our mask (or shoes), people will see we have peace and trust God with our story, like the humble birth of His Son, the Christ.

Dear Lord, thank You for humbly being born into this messy world to save us from our brokenness. Thank You for being a Wonderful Counselor, Mighty God, Everlasting Father, and Prince of Peace in my life. Help me understand that any area of my life that is "out of order" has not yet come under Your Lordship. Amen.

week three

> **Journal:** Write about some of the messy parts of your life for which you need to seek help from the amazing Counselor and from others in your First Place 4 Health group.

WONDERFUL COUNSELOR
by Karen Porter

Day 7

Names mattered to the Jews. Children were named for the social or political situation in which they were born, or for their father or mother, or for the leader or king of the time. The meaning of the name of a child was often a prophecy as to what the child would become. There are more than 2,000 names and titles for Jesus in the Bible, but Isaiah concentrated on four titles when he predicted the birth of the Messiah.

The first name Isaiah gave was *Wonderful Counselor*. A counselor gives advice to help us find purpose and devises plans for a good future. Who better to be our counselor than God, who knows all about us and every moment of our lives? Paul asked, "Who knows enough to give him advice?" (Romans 11:34 NLT). Isaiah described the counselor as *wonderful*. He would be astonishing and incredible. As we are told in 1 Chronicles 16:24, "Publish his glorious deeds among the nations. Tell everyone about the amazing things he does" (NLT).

The second name Isaiah gave the child is *Mighty God*. The Hebrew word used for *God* in this verse is the same word used in Psalm 50:1: "The LORD, the Mighty One, is God, and he has spoken; he has summoned all humanity from where the sun rises to where it sets" (NLT).

The child would be incomparable. "To whom can you compare God? What image can you find to resemble him?" (Isaiah 40:18 NLT).

Isaiah also used the name *Everlasting Father* for the child who would be born. *Everlasting* is a never-ending forever. He has always been, He is now, and He will always be. He existed before the beginning and has no end. Isaiah also wrote about the Everlasting Father in 63:16 when he said, "You are our Redeemer from ages past" (NLT).

And as the only begotten Son of the Father, the child is the Prince, and His princely title is *Peace*. Understanding, harmony, and reconciliation are all part of the peace that Jesus gives us. Jesus said, "I am leaving you with a gift—peace of mind and heart. And the peace I give is a gift the world cannot give. So don't be troubled or afraid" (John 14:27 NLT). His peace is ours, because we believe in Him. The child of many names is our Savior and our Friend.

> *Dear Lord, thank You for Your counsel when we don't know what to do. And thank You for Your control over all the world. You are our Father, and we love You. You are the Prince of Peace who gives us hope. You are wonderful and mighty and glorious. We praise You. Amen.*

Journal: List some things in your life today that need peace that can only come from Jesus.

Note
1. Lydia Saad, "Americans Plan on Spending a Lot More This Christmas," Gallup poll, November 16, 2015, http://www.gallup.com/poll/186620/americans-plan-spending-lot-christmas.aspx.

Group Prayer Requests

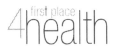

Today's Date: _____

Name	Request

Results

_____
_____
_____
_____
_____

Week Four

do not be afraid

SCRIPTURE MEMORY VERSE

An angel of the Lord appeared to them, and the glory of the Lord shone around them, and they were terrified. But the angel said to them, "Do not be afraid. I bring you good news that will cause great joy for all the people. Today in the town of David a Savior has been born to you; he is the Messiah, the Lord.

LUKE 2:9–11

WHAT CAN I GIVE HIM — Day 1
by Charlotte Davis

I am fifty years old, which means I have taken part in at least forty-five church Christmas programs. As the fifth child in a pastor's family, participation was never exactly optional. But I've always loved to worship God through singing, and I have continued to do so throughout my life. However, on December 6, 2015, I was beginning to wish I was not part of that year's Christmas musical at our church.

It was a dress rehearsal. If you have ever been part of a church worship team, you know these are often not what you could call "good" performances. A lot of time is spent working out all the kinks. This particular dress rehearsal, however, went beyond the usual challenges to being the most horrible one I can remember. First, the choir did not appear to even *know* the music, let alone be as familiar with it after three months of practices! I was designated the alto section leader (mainly because I am *loud* and they follow what I do, right or not), and I missed part after part. Unfortunately, the other sections were just as awful, missing notes and coming in at the wrong times. Actors missed line after line. Instrumentalists hit sour notes again and again. Our worship leader, normally a positive guy, looked frantic!

At one point in the rehearsal, the children's choir came into the sanctuary to practice with us. They bounced in, smiling and laughing. I leaned over to my alto friend, Judy, and whispered something like, "Well, maybe the cute factor of the kids will save us!" She responded with a hopeful nod, but with a far-from-convinced look on her face.

This particular musical included a not-as-familiar Christmas carol titled "In the Bleak Midwinter" by Christina Rossetti. As the choir sang the third verse, the children stood up and began acting out the nativity scene:

Angels and archangels may have gathered there,
Cherubim and seraphim thronged the air;
But His mother only, in her maiden bliss,
Worshiped the Beloved with a kiss.

Ella, an eight-year-old girl, had been assigned a solo for the last verse. Her young voice broke into these words, pure and innocent and sweet:

What can I give Him, poor as I am?
If I were a shepherd, I would bring a lamb;
If I were a Wise Man, I would do my part.
What can I give Him? Give Him my heart.

All the rustling and whispering silenced. Even the children were quiet as they listened closely to Ella's words and gazed at the manger scene. Tears filled my eyes. *This* was what Christmas was about, the reason we were even *doing* this program! We wrapped up the rehearsal that day, and when it came time for the final performances, God anointed our efforts with His Holy Spirit. Many said it was the best Christmas musical we had ever done.

Heavenly Father, help me to seek You first this Christmas season, giving You my full heart and attention, and not get distracted by things that don't really matter. Help me to truly worship the Child in the manger who became the Savior of the world. Amen.

Journal: Write out the lyrics of a Christmas carol. You might even want to find an old hymnbook and choose one that is less familiar to you!

Day 2: DO IT AFRAID
by Becky Turner

Isn't it interesting that the glory of the Lord brought about fear in the shepherds? Fear in itself is not a bad thing—it is not a sin. It is a defense mechanism that heightens our awareness and places our minds and bodies on alert. The problem is when we allow fear to stop us—to paralyze us. The fear of rejection stops us from asking someone out. The fear of hurt stops us from loving deeply. The fear of judgment stops us from confessing our greatest temptations or sins. The fear of failure stops us from pursuing our goals.

One First Place 4 Health participant I know lost more than 170 pounds. To all outsiders she appeared to be free from the bondage of food, but the truth was that she was scared. She feared that if she ever deviated from her "plan" for even a meal, she would gain all the weight back. This did not bring great joy in her life, nor did it allow the Savior to be all that He could be to her. She had to face her fear—*do it afraid*—and have chips and salsa (just not every night), enjoy an occasional dessert (but not the entire pie), and trust the Power who raised her Savior from the ground and now lived in her to help her walk in freedom to food.

This Christmas season, ask the Holy Spirit to grant you the power to make wise choices and practice self-control with every meal. Do not allow fear to stop you from going to the neighborhood Christmas party because you may eat too much or because you do not know how to track each bite. Also, do not allow fear of rejection stop you from asking for prayer from your fellow First Placers as you step out and trust Christ to be strong in your weakness. And if you make poor choices, do not allow fear of condemnation stop you from confessing that to another trusted friend and get back on track immediately.

When the glory of the Lord rises up in you and you *do it afraid*, His great joy will flood your soul.

> *God, Your power in me is greater than my fears. Increase my trust in You and grant me the wisdom to know how to access that power on a bite-by-bite basis. Amen.*

Journal: Write out three fears you have, and then find three Scripture references to help you overcome those fears.

Day 3 — FINDING JOY
by Helen Baratta

Living an overflowing life during the holidays threatens our joy. Irritability grows as we dwell on the concerns, robbing time with God and our self-care. Jesus said, "The worries of this life . . . choke the word, making it unfruitful" (Mark 4:19). Our circumstances begin capturing our thoughts.

The mopey people with whom we interact threaten our joy. We ourselves may sap joy, dimming the light of another. Jesus said, "Love one another. As I have loved you, so you must love one another" (John 13:34). God loved us and sent a Savior. God's gift, our Savior born, provides the solution. As the angel exclaimed years ago, we too must reach out and share the good news of God's great joy.

A desire for material things consumes our focus. We create wish lists and scrutinize the gifts we selected for others. We transform and perfect decorations and improvements, striving for the perfect holiday home. Jesus warned, "Do not store up for yourselves treasures on earth" (Matthew 6:19), but instead focus on treasures in heaven. "For where your treasure is, there your heart will be also" (verse 21). So, how do we find **JOY**?

Just look to Jesus. "Fixing our eyes on Jesus, the pioneer and perfecter of faith. For the joy set before him endured the cross, scorning its shame, and sat down at the right hand of the throne of God" (Hebrews 12:2). Jesus is our source of joy.

Obey our Lord. Jesus shared, "If you keep my commands, you will remain in my love . . . so that my joy may be in you and that your joy may be complete" (John 15:10–11). Complete joy flourishes when we obey.

Yearn for Jesus. "My soul yearns, even faints, for the courts of the Lord; my heart and my flesh cry out for the living God" (Psalm 84:2). When Jesus is our first desire, we yearn for nothing else. Jesus said, "But seek first [God's] kingdom and his righteousness, and all these things will be given to you as well." Including joy.

Lord, forgive me when I rush into Your presence, rattle off my wants, and scurry off to complete the tasks on my list. Help me yearn for Your presence, spend time sharing my thoughts, and then listen to Your desires too. Lord, fill me with Your joy. Amen.

> **Journal:** Write about a joy buster that you are struggling with today: a circumstance, a person, or a thing. How can you allow Jesus to introduce His joy to you?

A NEW PURPOSE
by Desiree Glass

Day 4

My mother started repurposing long before it was cool. In fact, at times I thought her repurposing was *uncool*. Why couldn't she just buy gift tags for our Christmas gifts instead of making her own out of last year's Christmas cards?

But when money got tight, some of Mom's frugality rubbed off on me. Besides, I couldn't bear to throw out my beautiful Christmas cards. Some of them were marvelous works of art—glittery winter scenes, colorful wildlife, bright shining stars, whimsical gingerbread men, cutesy snow people, awe-inspiring nativity scenes, and, of course, the radiant face of the Christ child. Each was unique, yet they carried the same message of hope, peace, and joy.

It seemed wrong to pitch something so beautiful. Shouldn't their purpose extend beyond a few short weeks? I soon found myself crafting my own gift tags from last year's Christmas cards. I cut off the front of the cards and attached them to packages and recycled gift bags. I smiled when a newly crafted tag matched the bag. I smiled when I realized I'd turned into my mother.

An angel brought the first Christmas greeting, the good news of the Savior. In turn, shepherds spread the word about what they had been told. Now we, as Christians, are sent, like Christmas cards, to continue spreading the word and tell of the love of God. In 1 John 4:9 we read that He was "made manifest among us, that God sent his only Son into the world, so that we might live through him" (ESV). Through Him, we have the gift of eternal life. Through Him, our lives are changed. Through Him, we have newfound purpose.

Each of us is a marvelously unique work of art (see Psalm 139:14), set apart as a vessel of honor for the Master's use (see 2 Timothy 2:21). Some of us glitter, some of us shine, but all of us have been designed to share the good news of Christ. How? By allowing the Father to rub off on us. "For it is God who works in you to will and to act in order to fulfill his good purpose" (Philippians 2:13).

It is God who changes us to share His message that never changes. He put His Spirit in our hearts at salvation as a deposit on His gift of eternal life (see 2 Corinthians 1:22). His Spirit will inspire us and give us the power to witness (see Acts 1:8). Our recycled lives will be like a letter from Christ (see 2 Corinthians 3:3), a gift tag beckoning others to open the gift as well. And that will be *very* cool.

Thank You, God, for Your indescribable gift! Thank You for changing my life and giving me new purpose. May I be a vessel of honor for Your use. Fashion me as You see fit so I may reach others with the message of Christmas. Amen.

Journal: Write three ways you can creatively share the message of Christmas.

do not be afraid

Day 5: GOOD NEWS
by Vicki Heath

I don't blame the shepherds. I would have been afraid too. Angels showing up all around in the dark of the night in the middle of nowhere would have been frightening. And I'm sure that seeing God's glory lighting up the sky would have been pretty spectacular. But then the God of all comfort had the angels say just the right words: "Do not be afraid. I bring you good news" (Luke 2:10). Good news! The world needs some good news.

On this night, the coming of the Messiah was the "good news that will cause great joy for all the people." The *people* included the inhabitants of Israel in that day and you and me in this day. Jesus embodies all of the good news we could ever need for any life situation. Regardless of our worries and problems, He doesn't just have the answer—He *is* the answer!

Do you need the good news that forgiveness can happen in families? Do you need the good news that God will be there to help you multiply the fishes and the loaves? Last Christmas, the best news was hearing from God, "Vicki, you are not to gain any weight over the holidays." This good news actually came to me in a miracle—my First Place 4 Health class decided to meet all through the holidays and not take a break. We met every Tuesday morning from November until the middle of January.

Good news! Not only did our group not gain weight, but we also lost weight! Deciding to not take a break kept us focused on the commitments we had made together earlier in the year. One of those commitments was to make every day a First Place 4 Health day. And as we did, Christ was glorified in our bodies as well as our spirits.

> *Dear Lord, because of You I have nothing to fear. You are the good news not only for me but also for all people. Help me to receive Your good news with great joy. Amen.*

Journal: Write about the good news you need to hear from God this Christmas. Seek the Christ of Christmas for the answers. Do not be afraid. Jesus is the good news, and He brings great joy!

Day 6
GOD IS FAITHFUL
by Sherry Leggett

I grab a tissue for the pending tears as the scene unfolds on Christmas Eve in the 1944 musical *Meet Me in St. Louis*. Judy Garland's character, Esther, sings the familiar ballad "Have Yourself a Merry Little Christmas" to cheer up her sister, Tootie, played by Margaret O'Brien. Esther and her family are distraught by their father's plans to accept a promotion in New York City, for it means they will have to leave behind their beloved home in St. Louis.

Just as music can evoke memories (as Judy's song always does for me), so can certain foods. In addition, the sense of smell is a direct path to the brain. Even the smell of a certain holiday dish can evoke an emotional response that ultimately sends us back to that holiday buffet more times than we even realize—and we don't even know why.

We can eat in response to feelings. Just like this ballad in the movie, the holidays can drum up a whole treasure chest of feelings, both good and bad. It's okay to have the emotion and think about the memory. We just can't bring back the good times or cover up the bad times with three slices of pecan pie or whatever is our holiday dish of choice.

If you are berating yourself over a bad food choice, stop the spiral of self-hate and own up to your feelings. Say to yourself, *I wish I hadn't eaten three pieces of pecan pie, but what is done is done. What can I do differently the next time I'm in that situation?* Focus on how you will eat well the next meal or day. Do not be afraid of the emotions or temptation. In 1 Corinthians 10:13, Paul states, "No temptation has overtaken you except what is common to mankind. And God is faithful; he will not let you be tempted beyond what you can bear. But when you are tempted, he will also provide a way out so that you can endure it."

Our First Place 4 Health group takes a moment before the holidays to think about what role holiday foods play in our memory banks. We plan our holiday plates to help us overcome the temptation to overeat. We use our food log in our Bible studies to log our food *prior* to the parties. We also plan our healthy snacks throughout the days leading up to the parties. By doing this, we know we are less likely to overindulge.

Dear Lord, thank You for being the great Messiah! Thank You for helping me conquer any temptation. Amen.

Journal: As you look forward to the upcoming season, think about what parties and events you need to plan your plate for to avoid over abundance. Write your plan below.

week four

THE BEST JOY
by Karen Porter

Day 7

A baby announcement! Proud parents pick out the most clever and colorful graphics to tell their friends and family the news. Some families hold extravagant "gender reveal" parties to proclaim a boy or girl. And when the baby is born, there are presents and parties with photos and videos and postings on social media. Families rejoice, grandmothers coo, and young moms and dads feel a bit overwhelmed.

When God announced the arrival of His Son, He sent an angel. But He didn't send the angel to the famous people or the important scribes and priests. Instead, the angel of almighty God announced the birth of the Savior of the world to a group of anonymous shepherds on a hillside. Shepherds were workers who rarely came to the crowded cities. Their work made them ceremonially unclean, so they weren't welcome in the temple. They were typically poor, and even outcasts, yet God proclaimed the good news to them.

Christmas—Jesus—is for every person, rich or poor, large or small, important or lowly. The worldwide gospel is the good news of great joy for all people. Jesus came to fill our greatest need: forgiveness and salvation. As Paul wrote, "You know the generous grace of our Lord Jesus Christ. Though he was rich, yet for your sakes he became poor, so that by his poverty he could make you rich" (2 Corinthians 8:9 NLT). Jesus' sacrifice was tremendous. He left the splendor of heaven, came to earth to live as a servant, and eventually died the worst kind of death on a cross—because of you (see Philippians 2:6–8).

Notice the great angelic announcement in Luke 2:11: "Today in the town of David a Savior has been born to you; he is the Messiah, the Lord." Scholars agree that these words are the beginning of the high point of redemptive history—the greatest moment in the history of the world. A Savior. The One. The Messiah. He would take the punishment for your sin and mine. The punishment meant death for Him, but payment in full for us. And because the debt of sin was paid, God forgives us.

To hear and receive the gospel is the highest and best joy. The angels said the good news would bring great joy. The word *joy* literally means laughter. Peter said the joy of the Lord is inexpressible (see 1 Peter 1:8). And all because a baby was born.

Dear Lord, thank You for announcing the good news of Jesus' birth to ordinary people, signifying that the good news of the gospel is for all people. We are grateful for Jesus, the Savior of the world. Amen.

Journal: Do you believe that Jesus came to forgive you? Journal some things that you feel you need to accept that forgiveness, and then let them go.

do not be afraid

Group Prayer Requests

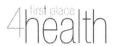

Today's Date: _____

Name	Request

Results

_____
_____
_____
_____
_____

Week Five

a new creation

SCRIPTURE MEMORY VERSE
Therefore, if anyone is in Christ, the new creation has come: The old has gone, the new is here!
2 CORINTHIANS 5:17

CHRISTMAS GIFTS
by Judy Marshall

Day 1

New years come on the heels of old ones. Excitement of New Year's Eve celebrations and making resolutions wanes within the first month of the new year. This happens because daily life is hard and monotonous . . . no longer a festive party. For days, weeks, months, we attempt by our own strength to force the changes required in our resolutions. This year's resolutions aren't actually new at all. We rearrange the words, hoping to gain control of the recurring habit we meant to change years ago.

Hear me—we don't need a change; we need a *transformation*!

In his book *Faith & Fat Loss,* Ron Williams writes, "True transformation begins with acknowledging your need for God." He compares spiritual and physical transformation to the caterpillar's becoming a butterfly. A change takes place, but the difference is a completely new creation. Williams adds, "If you only change, you have the ability to go back to the old way of life and to the old you, but once transformed you no longer have the ability to be who or what you once were. True transformation can only happen in the presence of a power that is much greater than man has to offer—this can only happen through the power of God."

Williams points out that going our own way in our own strength, using our own intellect, reasoning, and self-will, will lead to failure. Why else would we rephrase our New Year's resolutions and First Place 4 Health goals each year? We're trying to change rather than be transformed. We are losing the battle of weight loss because we accept self-indulgence, instant gratification, and gluttony. Williams reminds us, "We are trying to be effective against a problem that can only be fought and won through God's power. We must realize that the epidemic of being overweight and obese is a powerful tool the adversary is using to defeat God's people by causing us to be ineffective, depressed, without energy, sick [and] diseased."[1]

After rereading the previous words, I'm rewriting new goals for old habits I want God to transform into healthy habits:

1. *Portion size*: My prayer before I eat will be for God to remind me that He is my portion and for Him to help me choose to be satisfied *in Him* and with smaller servings.

2. *Balanced meals*: My prayer before I plan daily meals will be for God to remind me of the balanced food plan in First Place 4 Health and give me the desire for the healthiest choices.

3. *Exercise:* My prayer before I walk will be to offer thanks to God for the ability and safety to walk, to remind me to enjoy His creation, and to use my walk to listen for Him.

Join me . . . out with the old, in with the new! We want to be *transformed*!

> *Lord, I ask You to transform my mind and cause me to desire wise, healthy choices. Transform my self-indulgence into Spirit-control, instant gratification into patience, and gluttony into satisfaction. Amen.*

Journal: Rewrite your goals as a prayer that reflects your desire to be transformed rather than changed.

Day 2: A RESOLUTION FOR LIFE
by Delilah Dirksen

During a recent physical exam at my doctor's office, the nurse commented, "Delilah, your weight is remarkable." I was puzzled by this comment, because I still had some weight to lose. "Why is *my* weight remarkable?" I asked. She replied, "Because every year it stays the same."

Given our country's weight crisis, I don't know why it never occurred to me that most Americans' weight does not stay the same when they visit the doctor—and that maintaining the same weight is remarkable. It should come as no surprise that weight loss and exercise are topping the list of New Year's resolutions people make in America. They're also topping the list of resolutions people fail to keep. There's even a holiday to commemorate it. *Ditch New Year's Resolution Day* is not a Federal holiday but a holiday nevertheless, celebrated on January 17. It is observed as the most common day resolution-makers become resolution-breakers.

Statistics and science reports lend some explanation as to why people give in. According to a Barna survey, one of the reasons people struggle with keeping their resolutions is because they try to achieve personal change on their own.[2] *Psychology Today* cites a study by Baumeister, Vohs, and Tice that reports, "Your willpower, or what scientists refer to as self-control, is a very limited resource—and once it is used up, your ability to stick with your goals and resist temptation is threatened."[3]

So, how do we sustain our self-control beyond seventeen days? With enthusiasm! Did you know that the word *enthusiasm* means "in God"? It comes from two Greek words, *en,* which means "in," and *theos,* which means "God." Paul wrote, "When you believed, you were marked *in him* with a seal, the promised Holy Spirit" (Ephesians 1:13, emphasis added). One of the fruit of the Spirit is self-control (see Galatians 5:22), which does not expire because God does not expire. He is the "eternal King" (Jeremiah 10:10). Willpower is limited, but God's power is limitless.

I've been maintaining my weight loss since 2002 by practicing disciplines I learned through First Place 4 Health. I know that when I make mistakes, the old is gone and every second presents an opportunity for a new beginning. I do not have to do it alone—I have the help of God and a supportive community of friends to help me make the right choices for health emotionally, mentally, spiritually, and physically.

Together in Christ, we have an unsurpassed stick-to-it-ness that we can't sustain on our own. In the past, I reluctantly accepted I needed to be a First Place 4 Health *lifer.* This year, I *enthusiastically* renew my resolution: I'm *in* for life! It's a resolution for life—for both now and eternity. Are you *in*?

Lord, thank You for new beginnings. Help me to make necessary changes, plans, and wise choices to live my life in Your incomparably great power through Your Spirit in my inner being. I can do all things through You who gives me the strength. Amen.

Journal: "Sometimes we have to *let go and let God,* and other times we need to *get go, and get God.*"[4] Write about what you need to *let go* of to make your health a priority this year and what area of your First Place 4 Health plan you need to *get go*-ing on.

week five

NEW CREATIONS
by Susan Sowell

Day 3

Sometimes it helps to hear the story of someone who wrestles with the same thing that wars within our own heart. *Wrestle* and *war* are words that describe a battle. I'm not a fan of battle scenes. I don't like war movies, unless they are from less-harmful characters like Cinderella and her evil step-mother. The eyes of my heart crave peace, beauty, and happy endings. Those are the types of movies I like to watch. Yet while it works to skip out on movies with harsh battle scenes, it is inescapable for us to skip out on the harsh battle scenes in the war for our hearts.

It doesn't take convincing to see that the battleground we stepped onto from birth is far from the fairy-tale scenes we see in Disney movies. The battle we fight is real, and it is intended to capture our hearts. I knew about this type of battle long before I understood what it was about. At times, I felt the pierce of unseen arrows causing my heart to fear. At other times, I felt the arrows of shame, hopelessness, or depression cause my heart to sink into an unseen pit of despair. The scene is not one that any of us can skip by changing the channel, pretending it doesn't exist, and then expecting to experience victory in our lives.

In 2 Corinthians 5:17, Paul tells us who we are in the battle. We are covered by the blood of Jesus, given new life, and are victorious through the power of Christ! He won the battle for our hearts, and we belong to Him. Yes, the arrows will continue to come. Sometimes we will have our defenses down and will feel them pierce us. But that does not change the battle scene, for that scene has already been written. Nothing we do or don't do can change the script. The story for us as new creations in Christ was written at the cross in the blood of Jesus. It is the ultimate ending to the greatest story ever written.

As you begin this new year or new day, recognize it is an opportunity to choose how you view the character in your life story. The enemy will fire his arrows at you, attempting to capture your heart through food or any other trap that works for him. Those arrows will hurt your heart, so be aware of their presence in your pits of despair and shame. For you to experience victory on the battlefield, you must view yourself through the cross. The cross changed who you are in your life story and made you a new creation in Christ.

> *Thank You, Lord, for rescuing me from the enemy and giving me new life. Heal my heart of the pain the arrows have caused me and make me whole. I choose to believe what You say about me—that I am a new creation in You—and stand in victory on the battlefield. Amen.*

Journal: List some of the arrows you may face this holiday season. Now list God's truths that you can use against them.

MOVING FORWARD
by Barb Lukies

Day 4

This week's verse says to me, "Move forward to a new chapter." God has the chapters and pages already worked out. We just need to turn the page and see what's new.

My daughter will get married this month and have a new life ahead of her. It is an honor to see her grow into a mature Christian woman who has chosen a godly husband. They love God, and it is their desire to serve Him. Weddings come with expectations: the engagement, the planning of the wedding, and the planning ahead for the future. So many couples focus on the marriage ceremony and not the actual marriage itself. Marriage comes with letting go of the old self and moving ahead with a new life in Christ.

My husband and I have been married twenty-five years this new year. We have been through good times and hard times, healthy times and times of illness. It takes a lot of hard work, commitment, and communication, along with lots of prayer, for a marriage to last this long. It takes a daily working out of spiritual commitments, Bible study, and quiet time. It takes praying and learning Scripture to keep us on the right path.

I have been chronically sick for ten years. This has meant that I am unable to do things I could previously do. My husband and I are in a new era of our lives, with our children now adults and moving forward with their own lives. So we decided to attend counseling to learn a new way to communicate, create new goals, and re-establish a new future together.

We were committed to making our marriage work, and we have had to embrace new expectations of new things to come. The old has gone, and we now embrace the new life that God has planned for us. God gives us hope, and we know that we could not have made it on our own without Him. Change is never easy, no matter what your age. Some embrace it and look forward to a new start. Some cringe and don't want to change, but they know that in order to move forward, they must make changes— or they will stay in the same rut.

When we look to Christ, we find He has given us the example: embrace God, put on His mind, and lean on the Holy Spirit. He will show us the new direction He wants us to take.

Lord, help me to look to Your example and embrace all You have for my future. Amen.

Journal: Write about what parts of your old self God is asking you to leave behind. What are you looking forward to with excitement and anticipation for your new future life with Christ?

a new creation

Day 5: FRESH FOOTPRINTS
by Beverly LaHote Schwind

In January, a glistening snow in Tennessee covered the ground, trees, and rooftops. It looked as if a white carpet had been laid across the ground, and the trees dazzled like the artificial snow put on the Christmas trees the previous month. The earth felt peaceful and clean.

I woke up in the middle of one night and fixed myself a cup of chamomile tea. I turned on the outside lights and looked out the window. It was not snowing now, and I noticed many tracks in the snow. I went from window to window to see more and more tracks—different sizes. I could easily recognize the deer and the rabbit tracks, but there were others scattered here and there that I could not identify. I could tell there had been plenty of activity around our house in the early morning hours. I drank my tea and went to bed.

The next morning, I was eager to see if there were any more night signs of activity. But there was a fresh snowfall on the ground, and all the night tracks had been covered, never to be repeated in the same manner. It appeared the snow had been swept, and there was not one footprint visible.

This week's Bible verse says the old is gone. The new is here. If we have failed in the past at different challenges or have given in to temptations, we can start over. When we are in Christ, we have the strength of His Word to encourage us.

When I started my First Place 4 Health group, I was ten pounds heavier than I wanted to be. I started because some women I knew were having health issues—and their extra weight was adding to those issues. The program disciplined me and educated me in nutrition. I enjoyed the Bible study with the other women and the support system. I loved losing the ten pounds and keeping it off. Our group realized that when we backslid, our mistakes were forgotten and covered up, just like a fresh snowfall. The old was gone and the new was here.

My fresh footprints are behind me and will leave a temporary path others will see. They mark where I have been. I want my footprints to become a trail that others can follow as they walk with the Lord in all areas of their life. There are sugar addictions, eating disorders, drugs, and other distractions that can cause us to not reach a goal, but there is also the ability to start fresh and not let where we have been dictate where we are going. God will dust away the old footprints. We have a fresh path and a new year to begin.

Jesus, guide me in the new year to be a trail from which others may get encouragement and support. Help me to be strong and lead others in a walk with You. Keep me on the right path. Amen.

Journal: Think about an exercise, weight loss, or a Bible reading program that you started but ultimately gave up. Write about what you will do to start over, knowing that a new year for you starts when you begin.

Day 6: STARTING WITH THE NEW
by Karen Porter

Ever since I was a kid, I have loved a blank page and a sharpened pencil. Back then, I drew pictures and practiced my writing skills. Today I feel a wonderful thrill when I start a new journal or notebook. I like it so much that my shelves are full of half-full journals, each one with dozens of empty pages at the end. I simply can't wait to start over.

Imagine the possibilities of a fresh new book with untouched pages waiting for rich, beautiful words. I write new goals, new lists, new thoughts, and notes. I carefully copy meaningful Bible verses and then pencil in quotes that inspire me. It's such fun to start anew. I feel the same sensation when I open a new First Place 4 Health Bible study book—a new book, blank lines, and a new chance to follow Jesus to a balanced life.

Jesus understood the human need to start over. He told a man named Nicodemus that he had to be born again. The man didn't get it, saying that would be physically impossible (see John 3:1–4). But Jesus offered much more than physical change. He presented abundant life on earth and a kingdom for eternity. To start over for Jesus meant to turn away from sin and begin in a fresh new way.

It's hard to imagine how we can start over on a new wellness journey when we see the extra pounds on the scales or feel exhausted when we try to exercise. Discouragement overwhelms us. *I have too many pounds to lose. I have stiff joints. I eat because I'm unhappy. If you knew my past life, you'd understand. I can't.*

Paul said in 2 Corinthians 5:17 to put the old behind and see the new before. Sure we've made bad choices in the past—eating too much, sitting on the couch too long. But God says to turn the page and see the possibilities with the new day, the new week, the new year ahead.

Like me, you may wonder how to put away all those terrible mistakes, choices, and actions of the past. It is a good question. The answer is the love and mercy of Jesus. He knows how weak we are. He loves us anyway. He sees our poor choices and how we are mired in the consequences of our mistakes. He offers mercy no matter how many times we need to start over. "The steadfast love of the LORD never ceases; his mercies never come to an end; they are new every morning, great is your faithfulness" (Lamentations 3:22–23 ESV).

> *Lord, thank You for loving me and for showering Your mercy on me when I don't deserve it. Help me to see today as a new page in a journal. Help me record a day of good choices of healthy food, intentional exercise, Bible reading, prayer, and strong emotional relationships. Amen.*

week five

> **Journal:** Put the old behind and list some new choices you are going to make this week.

TAKE ACTION
by Sherry Leggett

Day 7

Nicodemus, a prominent leader among the Jews, went to Jesus late one night and asked, "Rabbi, we all know you're a teacher straight from God. No one could do all the God-pointing, God-revealing acts you do if God weren't in on it" (John 3:2 MSG). But the still-doubting Nicodemus asked more questions. Jesus eventually responded, "Instead of facing the evidence and accepting it, you procrastinate with questions. If I tell you things that are plain as the hand before your face and you don't believe me, what use is there in telling you of things you can't see, the things of God?" (John 3:11–12 MSG).

Wow, those are strong words from Jesus! I know the Spirit uses strong words with me to get me to remove my excuses to draw closer to Him through my wellness journey. How many times do we hear the Spirit talking to us and prompting us to take action, but we only see the limitations preventing us from accepting change?

"I just won't log this treat, so it won't count."

"How can I exercise? I don't have money for a gym membership."

"How can I pray when I don't have a room in my house for that?"

Jesus went on to give the famous line, "God so loved the world that he gave his one and only Son" (John 3:16). He added, "God didn't go to all the trouble of sending his Son merely to point an accusing finger, telling the world how bad it was. He came to help, to put the world right again" (verse 17 MSG). Jesus came to help us with our unhealthy habits. He came to bring down the behavior between us and God so we could fulfill His purpose.

Paul tells us in 2 Corinthians 5:17 that if we are in Christ, the old has gone and the new is here. God loves us too much to allow us to stay in the same rut. If we continue on a road we are currently living in without Christ—pleasing ourselves and procrastinating—it will only be unproductive. This journey to God's purpose isn't easy; it's full of starts, stops, and detours. The miraculous product in our lives will show God and be a testimony to His power. Change with God comes with His blessing.

Lord, thank You for your patience with me when I doubt and ask questions like Nicodemus! Help me to act on Your purpose that You present to me. Amen.

Journal: Write about what Jesus is calling you to change this year and how the habits in your life reflect Him. If you are you practicing a sin and looking for ways to justify it, seek the power of the Holy Spirit, flee from those desires, and talk to other Christians.

Notes
1. Ron Williams, *Faith & Fat Loss* (Salt Lake City, UT: RTW Publishing International, LLC, 2008), pp. 5–7, 23–24.
2. "Individualism Shines Through Americans' 2011 New Year's Resolutions," Barna, January 3, 2011, https://www.barna.org/barna-update/culture/465-americans-resolutions-for-2011#.Vxl90mN0aYU.
3. R.F. Baumeister, K.D. Vohs, and D.M. Tice, "The Strength Model of Self-Control," *Current Directions in Psychological Science,* 2007, vol. 16, no. 6, pp. 537–547.
4. Saying from Dr. Jeffrey Louis Hansis (1949–2008).

Group Prayer Requests

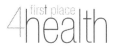

Today's Date: _____

Name	Request

Results

_____
_____
_____
_____
_____

Week Six

making a new way

Scripture Memory Verse
See, I am doing a new thing! Now it springs up; do you not perceive it? I am making a way in the wilderness and streams in the wasteland.
Isaiah 43:19

A PROMISE
by Martha Rogers

Day 1

This week's verse is a promise—a matter-of-fact statement of what God is doing for you. This is the first day of the rest of your life. Jesus is ready to do something new in you. He is making a way for you into the new year and a new beginning for a closer relationship with Him. What happened last year is past, today is the present, and tomorrow is your future. Live today with Him and look to the future where you will spend eternity. Let His love be a wellspring in your heart and soul.

When you look to the future, God prepares the way for you. So instead of resolutions this year, think of ways you can serve Him and strengthen your relationship with Him. Your First Place 4 Health Bible study gives you a place to start to search the Bible and find those "streams in the wasteland." Nothing can be done about the past or can change it. But we have today to live for Christ and do His work as we look to the future and what it will bring.

Your service as a Christian is to let that "new thing" spring up in you as you read God's Word, pray, and give thanks. Forget past rejections, disappointments, failures, and troubles, and concentrate on what He is making new in your life this year. Even as you go through deep waters of financial difficulties, illnesses, family problems, and career detours, you are in God's hands. Call on Him to help you through this day and show you the "new thing" He has for you. He will make a way in that wilderness and lead you to new heights of spiritual joy.

Remember that none of us have a claim on a great future. It may look wonderful today, but one moment can change everything and alter what happens from here on. Only God's joy, His strength, and His streams in the wasteland will see you through. So look to Him for guidance as you seek your way through the wilderness of life. Rejoice and be glad in today, count the blessings He has given (even when they seem so few), press on toward the future and your high calling (which draws you heavenward), trust Him to take care of the future, and stand firm in your belief of His promise for new things He will do in your life.

Heavenly Father, help us to live today as You would have us live. Give us the courage and stamina to press on even when we would rather give up. Help us to follow You and find those streams in the desert that will fill us with living water. Amen.

Journal: Make a list of things you can do for yourself and for God in the coming year, such as improving your relationship with Him or beginning a new healthy habit. Then list what new things He can do in your life.

making a new way

Day 2: MOMENT BY MOMENT
by Lauraine Snelling

Today I sit here whining. "Why, Lord, did I say I would write a devotional?" I don't write devotionals; I write stories. I just read the sample and am feeling a bit gut-punched. How can I work a story in here? After all, we learn by story—God created us this way. The Bible is a collection of stories. Jesus taught by story.

Hmmm. So, who is the character in this mini story? It's me and my "*Lord, I-can't-do-this*" attitude. This rebellion has all the earmarks of a spiritual disease. Wouldn't you know it, this week in Bible study we just read the story of the two sons in Matthew 21:28–32. The one son says "I'll do it" but doesn't, while the other says "no" and goes ahead and does the task. I said I'd do this, and so I will. Or rather, so I *am* doing it.

I turn to this week's verse in Isaiah 43:19 and read, "Behold I am doing a new thing." Stop right there. "Lord," I say, "You have the most incredible sense of humor. So, I get it. You—me—*we* are doing a new thing here." The verse continues, "Now it springs forth, do you not perceive it?" I focus on the word *now*. I agree with that; we are doing this now. I cannot put it off any longer. "I want to be obedient, Lord," I pray. "Thank You for promising to help."

I think back to other lessons. Our mighty Lord God promises to step in when we ask for help. Remember the Peter prayer? The one where he takes his eyes off Jesus when walking on the water and starts to sink? Peter cries out, "Lord, save me!" (Matthew 14:30).

Think on that most simple prayer: "Lord, help me!" Three little words—the panic prayer. Jesus didn't wait until the water closed over Peter's head to help. Instead, He *immediately* lifted Peter up, and probably even helped him back into the boat. Did Jesus scold and threaten Peter, even roll his eyes? No. But Peter got the lesson, I am sure. Just think if we cried, "Lord, help me!" before we began to sink? If we learned to rely on Him in the beginning? How much energy and time would we save? How much closer to Him would we feel?

Back to Isaiah. "I will make a way in the wilderness and rivers in the desert." Do you see the verb there? *Will.* Definitive. "I will make . . ." That wilderness could be my heart; He is making a way there. A way of obedience; of living up to my agreement. "And rivers in the desert." We so often are the desert where He promises "rivers of living water."

Lord, help me, moment by moment, that all I do will glorify You. I want to walk with You and seek Your face. I want to rejoice in the new things You begin and bring to completion with eyes to perceive them immediately. Thank You. Amen.

Journal: List some new things you will try and some current situations where you need to ask the Lord for help.

Day 3 — ENCOURAGING OTHERS
by Arla Frigstad

It was all about me and what I thought I needed. I had joined First Place 4 Health, at the urging of a friend, to find out about this new program at our church. I figured I'd lose one to two pounds a week and be "all done" in two to three sessions. Have you heard the saying, "We plan and God laughs?" I was foolishly relying on myself. That was more than five years ago.

God had a different idea and a different timeline. "See, I am doing a new thing!" God had a bigger picture than my limited view. He knew that I would learn and retain more if I stayed in the program longer. He knew there was much more I needed to learn—and it was much more than just losing weight.

Along the way, He also wanted me to understand that my actions affected not only me but also other members in my class. My actions affected others who might be thinking about the program and about the program itself. If I didn't do my homework and was not prepared, that attitude could spread to others. If I didn't follow the program, I was much less likely to find any success. And if I wasn't finding success, how would that encourage others to want to join? My choices could be responsible for others adopting a negative view of the program.

What you and I do *matters*. We are not living in a vacuum. Fortunately, when we ask God for help and direction, He has patience with us and gently guides us in the way He wants us to go. "Now it springs up; do you not perceive it?" God's way added years to my journey. That journey is still continuing, but it has been richer than I would have ever imagined. Along the way He has been growing me emotionally, physically, spiritually, and mentally. Had I lost the weight in the first year and quit, I would have missed out on so much.

"I am making a way in the wilderness and streams in the wasteland." If we surrender to God's will and His timing in our lives, we will be blessed beyond our original expectations for the First Place 4 Health program. Our dedication and good choices will encourage others in their journey . . . along the way.

Heavenly Father, I often think I know best and forge stubbornly ahead. Help me to rely on You more in this new year. And when I struggle, gently remind me that it is only with You that I will be successful, and pull me back to You. Amen.

Journal: Think about any area of your life that you are stubbornly holding onto and not giving up to God's control. Write down what steps you could take to put God in first place in that area.

Day 4: GOD WILL MAKE A WAY
by Lucinda Secrest McDowell

Throughout Yellowstone Park, visitors are constantly reminded by signs and official guides that they are in the wild, lest they forget and grow complacent with the beauty . . . and the creatures. Do you sometimes forget that life in today's culture is a lot like being "in the wild"? Unexpected threats can endanger our path if we let down our guard and forget to call on God for His strength and wisdom for the journey.

Perhaps that has happened to you. You started out tentatively, indulging in that potentially dangerous habit. A little bit can't hurt, can it? But then, as your poor choices continued, you discovered that you had been pulled into a "wild" situation with harmful consequences. Isaiah reminds us that God will make "a way in the wilderness." I love the praise song by Don Moen that proclaims, "He will make a way where there seems to be no way." That's exactly what our faithful and powerful God will do for you and me in the wilderness of our lives.

As the New Year begins, where do you need Him to make a way where there seems to be no way? A medical issue? Paying your bills? Reconciling with a loved one? Becoming healthier? Emotional wounds? Your work or need for work? Freedom from an addiction? Clarity on an important decision?

Friend, this is a new year, and God is "doing a new thing." You and I need no longer wander in the wilderness, fearful at every turn that we will be broadsided by problems we cannot solve. God promises to walk beside us and guide us through an unknown future. Yes, indeed, He will make a way. The question is, will we follow?

Heavenly Father, sometimes I am confused at which path to take and fearful that I will fail You and those depending on me. Help me to see this new year as a fresh opportunity to follow Your will and Your way. Amen.

> **Journal:** Write down your two greatest concerns as the new year begins. Now look up scriptural promises that speak to those issues. Rewrite the Scripture as a prayer to God. Continue to pray over these things until God clearly answers. Then remember to thank Him.

week six

HE WILL MAKE A WAY
by Desiree Glass

Day 5

If you knew me like my First Place 4 Health friends do, you would know of my dream to publish my book, *The Prettiest Sight to See: A Story of the Holly Wreath*. Our small group of ladies, having regularly shared with each other the most intimate details of our lives, have grown quite close. Since the end of our twelve-week session coincided with Christmas, we felt a holiday victory celebration was in order.

As I was arranging the food table, I couldn't help but hear the whispering among the ladies. *They have something up their sleeve*, I thought. When a couple of them slipped away, I was sure of my suspicion. A rustling at the door soon caught my attention, and my breath caught in my throat when I turned to see two of them enter with a beautiful berry-laden holly bush. They placed it right in front of me and said, "Plant it someplace where you will see it every day—so your dream will always be in sight."

So I did—right alongside my driveway. As I knelt to pat the earth firmly in place around my new plant, I breathed a quick prayer for a fruitful harvest. I then positioned in front of the holly a yard ornament emblazoned with the word *believe*. Every day, without fail, I turned my eyes toward the shrub as I passed by, believing in my heart that my prayer would be answered.

But one day I gasped when I saw nothing but a stand of scraggly brown sticks. *What happened? Did I not water it enough? What does this mean, God?* I had heard a sermon about dreams and how those that aren't watered will wither and die. *Had I not worked hard enough? Was the death of the holly a sign—or a natural consequence of physical drought?*

I was afraid to share the bad news with my friends, so instead I picked up a new holly from the local nursery to replace it. But where would I plant it? Would planting the new holly in the same place where the original holly had died be a good idea? As I inspected the spot, my eyes grew wide with surprise. Shiny new leaves had sprung forth at the base of the plant and encircled the dead uprights like a wreath. *My holly isn't dead after all!* I thought. *And neither is my dream. Forgive me, Lord, for doubting. Thank You for reviving the holly and renewing my hope. I trust You to make my dream come true.*

We all experience those seasons of drought where our lives appear stagnant. Our dreams haven't materialized, and we start to doubt. Let us remember that God will make a way in His perfect timing. And maybe this will be the year.

> *Lord, You are like an evergreen tree, yielding Your fruit to me throughout the year (see Hosea 14:8). I can't wait to see the new things You have in store! Amen.*

Journal: Write out one of your dreams and identify something you can do today to move you closer to achieving it. Follow up with a prayer, believing that God will make a way for your dream to spring forth.

A NEW THING
by Marie Rascoe

Day 6

On the first day of this year, my husband and I set out on a trip to Florida. This was not just another vacation for us. Since both of us had retired, it was our first time to spend a couple of months near our son and his family. After months of researching, we had finally secured a rental just a few miles from them. A new thing!

As we rode along that day, we reflected on all that had happened in that year. We first recounted blessings from God. He had sent a new pastor to our church, we had celebrated forty-eight years of marriage, my husband had undergone a successful heart procedure, and we had completed a place of service in our church. We reflected on God's hand of mercy in our family members' lives, the home-going of my sister, and countless answers to prayers.

I recalled how the First Place 4 Health class at my church had experienced numerous blessings over the year. God had led us to trust Him by faith for new things as we journeyed along together. We had memorized Isaiah 43:18–19 earlier in the year, and I remembered prayer requests that group members had shared and trusted God for the outcome. It had been a special blessing to see God leading this entire First Place 4 Health ministry to some new things.

As my thoughts shifted to my personal journey of wellness, my mind wandered back to the first time, in 1991, that I attended a First Place 4 Health orientation. I was a full-time college student, teaching a Sunday school class and juggling a household. After hearing the nine commitments, I was overwhelmed. How could I add one more thing? God was certainly presenting *a new thing*!

My daughter and I joined together. She saw to it that we stayed on track. She was a great accountability partner—which I desperately needed. If it had not been for her persistence, I would have fallen by the wayside many times over. That first session, I lost twenty pounds. Truly, a new thing for me! But God was not finished. The next session, I was asked to lead a class. Except for a few detours, God has kept me in this ministry ever since.

More than once, I have heard Carole Lewis say, "I'm in it for the long haul." It is easy to get in a rut and allow ourselves to become complacent or comfortable, whether it is in leading or participating in a healthy lifestyle. How do we keep the freshness and the zeal to carry on? Isaiah 43:19 is the secret for success. It begins with *see*. In order to see, we must be looking. Are you looking for the new thing God is doing? Are you sometimes guilty, like me, of putting God in a box and expecting Him to work the same as He did last time? May we start out the year looking for the new thing God wants to do in and through us.

Now it springs up. This reminds me of the little crocus flowers that are among the first to bloom in the spring. Sometimes they even push their way through the last remains of winter snow as they spring up to announce that summer is on the way—a new thing!

I am making a way in the wilderness and streams in the wastelands. The word *wilderness* denotes a negative, challenging way. The children of Israel wandered for forty years in the wilderness because of their disobedience and rebellion toward God. In our journey to wellness we'll encounter wilderness times, but these can become springboards for learning important truths from God's Word. May we accept these challenging times, as well as the good times, to move us toward the new things God has in mind.

Lord, as I stand at the threshold of the new year, help me to be watchful and obedient as You make a way, even in the wilderness, for new things. Amen.

Journal: List some of the new things that God is calling you to do in the upcoming year.

Day 7 — TAKING THE FIRST STEPS
by Ramona Miller

Reading this week's verse reminds us of God's direction and provision. He gives us guidance as we navigate this thing called *life*. Often we've wandered for so long that it's hard to imagine a path out of the wilderness. Sometimes we lose hope we'll ever leave this desolate place. Too many times we come to a place where we feel this may be our lot in life.

The verse in Isaiah also speaks of streams in the wasteland, which is God's provision for us. "My God will meet all your needs according to the riches of his glory in Christ Jesus" (Philippians 4:19). The amazing fact about God is that He not only gives us necessities but also is "able to do immeasurably more than all we ask or imagine" (Ephesians 3:20). Without our knowledge God makes arrangements to meet our needs, supplying us with direction and provision from seemingly out of nowhere. Our job is to seek, trust, and follow His nudges.

There was a time when I felt as if I were wandering in the wilderness of life. I had been in this place so long, and it was hard to envision things being any different. My daughter had been suffering from a chronic health issue that had lasted for nearly eight years. Not only had I prayed for her many times, but many others had also prayed for her as well.

Then one winter day, God directed me to ask thirty women to pray for her for thirty days. Psalm 37:23 says, "The LORD directs the steps of the godly" (NLT), and this was definitely stepping out in faith for me. But I did it, and after the thirty days, my daughter was doing better. In the next six months, she was remarkably better. After more than two years, it's amazing to see what God has done in her life!

Not only did God give me direction on asking for prayer, but He also provided a great First Place 4 Health group that supported her on the journey toward balance. She was able to lose seventy-five pounds. That's not the end of the story, however; she's been able to maintain the weight loss for more than one and a half years. And there's a bigger miracle, for she is on a drug that has the highest weight gain for this category of medications. Her doctor can hardly believe she is able to maintain this weight loss, much less lose weight!

God will make a way in our wilderness, but we must choose to follow Him. When we take the first steps, even if they are hard, He will provide and continue to direct our paths.

God, help me to follow You and allow You to provide for my needs.
May I recognize Your direction for balance in every area of my life. Amen.

Journal: Write about an area in which you need God's direction, and then write a prayer giving Him control. Try to include promises in Scripture that remind you of His faithfulness.

making a new way

Group Prayer Requests

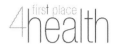

Today's Date: _____

Name	Request

Results

_____
_____
_____
_____
_____

A Joy-full Season
holiday survival tips

Maintaining healthy eating habits and an exercise regimen during the holidays can seem like an overwhelming task. Many times, all of our good habits that we have worked so hard to develop are thrown out the window as soon as November arrives! Planning ahead for holiday challenges is the key to surviving the holidays with those healthy habits intact. Following the suggestions in this section will help you experience a healthier holiday season.

PLAN AHEAD

- Find a holiday exercise buddy to walk with you daily or attend an aerobics class together. Make exercise a priority!

- Start a neighborhood tradition. Invite your neighbors to walk the neighborhood or community and sing Christmas carols along the way.

- Find healthy holiday recipes that will fit into the Live It Plan and that you will enjoy serving to holiday visitors.

- Focus on friends and family rather than on food. Make a special gift for each person attending your holiday get-together. Take digital group pictures and place a print in a Thanksgiving card for each person to take home with him or her as a keepsake.

SHOP SMART

- Park far away from the front door of the mall. Walk briskly, get some exercise, and save time looking for a parking space.

- Stop in the name of health! Don't even think of stopping for a treat at the food court. Pack some shopping snacks in your bag: yogurt, raisins, an apple, a banana, or pretzels. Planning ahead will prove to be a money saver and a calorie cutter.

- Warm up. Before actually making any purchases, take a stroll through the entire mall, and then go back to make purchases. This will not only add steps to your shopping day but will also help you make informed decisions about your purchases.

IT'S A PARTY

- Avoid the buffet table. Find someone to visit with who is sitting far away from the food. Focus on conversation, not on eating.

- Keep a glass of water or diet soda in your hands. This will help to keep your hands out of the high-calorie goodies.

- Bring a healthy appetizer like raw veggies or fruit to ensure that you will have something to snack on that supports your healthy habits.

THE PARTY'S OVER

- If you end up with leftovers that are tempting, send them home with your guests or share them with an elderly friend or family member.

- Freeze some of the leftovers in single servings to take for lunches or to have for dinners on the run.

- In preparation for the new year, purge your pantry of any junk foods or tempting foods. Out with the old, in with the new!

A NEW BEGINNING

- Greet the new year with a healthy attitude. Write one goal for the year in each of these areas: spiritual, emotional, mental, and physical.
- Start the new year off by planning your first week of menus along with your shopping list.
- Renew your subscriptions to any health newsletters or magazines for the coming year, or sign up to receive free health and fitness email newsletters or other publications.

HAVE A STRESS-FREE THANKSGIVING

- **Experiment:** Before the big day, experiment with recipes to familiarize yourself with their preparation. Get everything out on the counter and ready to go.
- **Prepare:** Prepare as much as possible in advance. For example, homemade cranberry sauce tastes better after curing in the refrigerator for a few days. Pre-measure seasonings and store them in labeled bags or containers. Clean, cut, and store vegetables in plastic bags in the refrigerator.
- **Enlist help:** Let your family set the table. Children will gobble up the chance to make place cards, fold napkins, and dress up the holiday table. This will keep them out of the kitchen while you attend to the food.
- **Serve buffet-style:** Use pretty serving bowls and silver utensils. Guests can help themselves to seconds whenever they want, while you remember your portion sizes.
- **Let the bird rest:** Let the turkey rest before slicing. To avoid a last-minute crunch and assure a tender turkey, let the bird rest out of the oven, covered, for about thirty minutes before slicing.
- **Microwave:** Use your microwave oven. Take advantage of this appliance to quickly reheat food before serving when all the burners on the stovetop are occupied.

HEALTHY HOLIDAY COOKING HINTS

- **Cut the fat:** Purchase a turkey without added fat—that is, a turkey that has butter or oil injected under the skin. If you use broth from the turkey, remove the fat. This can be done by allowing the broth to cool in the refrigerator or by skimming the broth with ice cubes.

- **Cut the cream:** Instead of using cream in your recipe, use fat-free Half-and-Half® or evaporated skim milk.

- **Experiment with dips:** The holiday season is a good time to experiment with dips. Use plain yogurt instead of sour cream. Even though the fat-free sour cream is devoid of fat grams, it is also devoid of nutrients. (Keep in mind that our goal in First Place 4 Health is to eat foods with as many nutrients as possible.)

- **Go with sugar-free pies:** Quick and easy pies can be made from instant or cook-and-serve sugar-free pudding. You can make any flavor fruit pie by using fresh fruit such as apples or peaches. Slice fruit, place in a saucepan, add a cup of apple juice (or other fruit juice) and one cup water, and cook until softened. Sweeten to taste with artificial sweetener. Add spices, if desired, and thicken with cornstarch. You now have a sugar-free, fat-free filling.

- **Substitute with applesauce:** Applesauce is a great substitute for fat and sugar in recipes. You can exchange a half cup of applesauce for a half cup of oil or for a half cup of sugar. (Note: substantial amounts of substitutes for the sugar and oil do not exchange well. That is why it is best to only replace part of the sugar or oil.)

- **Make a better frosting:** Use marshmallow fluff for frosting. Replacing the fat and sugar in the frosting with marshmallow achieves the perfect consistency with many fewer calories. Also, keep in mind that cutting sugar in half and adding a teaspoon of vanilla as a replacement can give just as much flavor with a lot less calories.

BRINGING JOY TO OTHERS

"And let us consider how we may spur one another on toward love and good deeds" (Hebrews 10:24).

- **Closet and toy clean out:** Have your children go through their toys and clothes and find some that they can donate to a second-hand store or a homeless shelter. Explain that for many parents, buying gifts for friends and family may be difficult, so this is a way to help those families. Have the kids decorate a large box to serve as a collection box.

- **Make greeting cards:** Kids love art projects, so this is a popular activity. Consider delivering cards to a local nursing or veteran's home. In addition to greeting cards, you can make Christmas decorations like paper chains or snowflakes, which are a great way to brighten what may be an otherwise dreary environment for people.

- **Help a neighbor:** Engage a team of friends to clandestinely rake leaves or shovel snow for an elderly neighbor for a whole month. Or volunteer to help a young mom by taking her young child for a stroller ride.

- **Help the hungry:** Donate food to a food bank this holiday season. Some families buy the same ingredients that they use for their holiday dinner and donate them to a food bank, which can make the experience more meaningful for a child. Better yet . . . when you drop off the donations, stay for a while and help pack boxes and sort food. (To find a food bank near you, go to Feeding America.)

- **A new kind of advent calendar:** Instead of candy, fill your calendar with ideas for activities and service projects.

- **Random acts of kindness:** A service project doesn't have to be a formal event organized through an established nonprofit organization. It's just about helping. Bring cookies and thank-you cards to your volunteer firefighters, police officers, or librarians. Make care kits for the homeless that include a bottle of water, a granola bar, and a $5 gift card to a local pharmacy. Leave change at a vending machine with a note that says: "Please Enjoy This Random Act of Kindness. Happy Holidays!"

- **Send Christmas notes:** Send Christmas notes to at least six people who blessed you this past year. For example, you could thank your First Place 4 Health leader or a member who has encouraged you. Be specific about how they helped you.

- **Invite someone to be part of your holiday:** Invite someone to be a part of your holiday celebration who would have little family activity otherwise. You could take that person to a church party or to look at Christmas lights.

- **Get spiritual:** Make a spiritual event part of your Christmas tradition. Read the Christmas story in Matthew 1:18–25, Luke 2:1–20, and Matthew 2:1–12, or attend a candlelight service or church pageant.

- **Tell stories of family Christmases past:** Find visual reminders such as old decorations, cards, photos, or gifts of past Christmases that you have experienced. Share stories that older relatives have told about their Christmases. Heirloom stories tie families to their heritage and encourage them to make memories for the future.

- **Slow down:** Slow down, take a deep breath, and plan a successful and meaningful holiday. Drop the unimportant, even if others pressure you to do those things. Add the important, even if no one but you finds meaning in them. Enjoy people more than things and the gift of the Son of God more than anything else! When He is in first place, all the season's events hold the potential for joy.

AVOID EMOTIONAL TRAPS

- **Comparison:** Festive outings can be occasions for being placed in uncomfortable situations that give rise to feelings of inferiority, embarrassment, or shame. This may occur at company dinners, family gatherings, or church parties where poise and physical appearance seem to be more important than ever. These situations may stir up past feelings of not measuring up that can date back to a childhood party or an embarrassing blunder in a Christmas play. When you begin to feel inferior or ashamed, it's time to remind yourself what God's Word says about you! Memorize Scripture verses that will arm you with truthful encouragement when you are tempted to compare.

- **Expectations:** For many people, the holidays are not emotional lifts but emotional downers. All the celebration makes tough times seem tougher and sad times seem sadder, often because people expect to be filled with joy. Sometimes we have idealized expectations for holiday events that are not based in reality, and when those expectations are not met, we become depressed. Learn to be realistic about your expectations, and don't punish yourself if you are having a difficult time. Draw close to God and ask Him to soothe your troubled spirit.

- **Difficult settings:** The time between Thanksgiving and New Year's Day draws more families together than at any other time. If family gatherings are affirming, they can be an emotionally positive time. But for millions of people, the holidays are filled with past pain, guilt, unresolved anger, destructive secrets, and old unhealthy patterns. Painful family situations include a divorced couple splitting Christmas with the children or an adult visiting an overly controlling mother, an alcoholic father, or an out-of-control sibling. In order to minimize the negative influence of holiday distractions to healthy living, it is important to increase the positive factors.

- **Evaluate:** Looking back on the past few holiday seasons, consider what caused you pain and what caused joy. Add more of the joy factors (for example, sponsoring a needy family or attending a Christmas Eve service). Attempt to discover patterns of pain, and make plans to minimize their impact before they occur (for example, keeping your visit short or putting off a visit until a less stressful time).

- **Plan and get support:** Don't just let the holidays sweep you along. Plan now what you will or won't do. Seek the support of at least two people to be your reality check and prayer-support partners. They can give their impression of what is a reasonable or healthy reaction to low self-esteem issues or painful family situations.

A Joy-full Season leader discussion guide

The First Place 4 Health holiday session is six weeks long (with one group meeting per week) and is recommended for any member who has completed at least one regular First Place 4 Health session. This shorter session is specially designed for First Place 4 Health members who desire to maintain their healthy habits during the holidays.

Each group meeting should last approximately one hour, with fifteen-minute segments set aside for (1) weigh-in and memory verse recitation, (2) Wellness Spotlight, (3) devotion/journal discussion, and (4) prayer requests and prayer. Before the first meeting, your group members should memorize the Week One memory verse as they read the daily devotions, do the journaling assignments, and complete the prayer partner form to turn in during the meeting. They should also fill out their Live It Tracker each day and turn it in at the group meeting. (See the *First Place 4 Health Leader's Guide* for tips on how to evaluate your members' Live It Trackers.)

Following is a suggested outline for each of the six group meetings.

WEEK ONE: WE GIVE THANKS
Weigh-in and Memory Verse (15 minutes)
Weigh and measure members and listen as they recite the week's Scripture memory verse.

Wellness Spotlight (15 minutes)

Staying motivated during the holidays can be especially difficult, but staying motivated can be difficult at any time of the year if one loses sight of how he or she can benefit from his or her weight-loss efforts. Ask members to share their answers to the following:

1. Have you ever gained weight during the holidays?
2. What tempts you to overeat?
3. What's the payoff when you overeat? What do you get out of overeating?
4. What might you gain by staying focused during the holidays?

Guide your members to make realistic goals for the holiday session. Have them discuss in small groups or with the whole group some strategies that may keep them focused on their holiday goals.

List these strategies on a whiteboard, chalkboard, or poster board. If they have not yet done so, have them complete the goal-making exercise in the introduction of this book.

Devotion/Journal Discussion (15 minutes)

Invite volunteers to share about losses they have experienced, and then list any blessings that have come from the loss.

Ask members to share Scripture verses that have brought comfort or healing to their lives.

Prayer Requests/Prayer (15 minutes)

Have members write a praise or something for which they are thankful on small index cards. Send a basket around and fill it with the blessings.

For the prayer time, read the praises, and then ask each member to pray by speaking a one-word praise (e.g., children, health, Jesus).

Before the group leaves, pass around the basket again for prayer partner forms. Have each member take a form from the basket on his or her way out.

WEEK TWO: OUR ANSWERS TO PRAYER

Weigh-in and Memory Verse (15 minutes)

Weigh and measure members and listen as they recite the week's Scripture memory verse.

Wellness Spotlight (15 minutes)

Each of your group members will certainly want to survive the holidays with his or her healthy habits still in place. So, for this session, you will begin to plan activities with your group that will take them through the holidays and enable them to become healthier physically, emotionally, mentally, and spiritually in the coming year.

Ask members to split into pairs and review the Holiday Survival Tips, selecting one activity for each week from the list. Have them write that activity on a specific date of their calendars, noting whether it is aimed at their physical, spiritual, emotional, or mental health.

Invite partners to pray for each other during the meeting about the activities they have chosen and to keep each other accountable in coming weeks.

Having your members anticipate challenges or obstacles that they will face on Thanksgiving will allow them time to develop strategies to overcome those challenges. Instruct members to write out what they plan to eat on Thanksgiving Day. Refer them to the Thanksgiving Day menu and to the recipes that follow, as well as to the "Stress-free Thanksgiving" section in the Holiday Survival Tips.

Ask members to share the strategies they plan to use to overcome some of the challenges that this holiday will bring. Again, refer them to Holiday Survival Tips for ideas.

Devotion/Journal Discussion (15 minutes)

Ask members to list character traits of God. Then have volunteers explain how they have come to know more fully a specific character trait of God.

Write Psalm 118:21 on a whiteboard, chalkboard or poster board, and display it in the room. Ask volunteers who have memorized the verse to quote it for the group. Then have each member tell one thing they are thankful to God for in their life.

Prayer Requests/Prayer (15 minutes)

Pray aloud in unison using Psalm 11:21, and then have volunteers pray and thank God for His wonderful works.

Before the group leaves, pass around the basket for prayer partner forms. Have each member draw a form from the basket on his or her way out.

WEEK THREE: TO US A SON IS GIVEN

Weigh-in and Memory Verse (15 minutes)

Weigh and measure members and listen as they recite the week's Scripture memory verse.

Wellness Spotlight (15 minutes)

Ask members to consider how focusing on giving to others can help them maintain their fitness goals. Refer them to the "Bringing Joy to Others" section in Holiday Survival Tips and lead a discussion about which ideas work for them and what things they might do to bring joy to their own community. Would doing it help to put the focus on Christ and others instead of self?

Devotion/Journal Discussion (15 minutes)

Before the meeting, call a member and ask him or her to prepare to give a brief (five to six minute) testimony of his or her salvation. Begin the devotion/journal discussion by inviting this member to share.

Ask members, "What is your focus during this holiday?" Invite volunteers to share how they (as an individual or as a family) keep their focus on the birth of Christ rather than on buying gifts.

Discuss all the roles that they take on, such as mom, dad, sister, wife, volunteer, Sunday School teacher, choir member, and so on during this busy season.

As a group, read Isaiah 9:6 aloud, and then list the names of Jesus that are stated in this verse. Ask members which name they need to call on to meet the needs of a specific responsibility that they must fulfill.

Prayer Requests/Prayer (15 minutes)
Invite members to pray aloud short prayers that use the names of Jesus found in Isaiah 9:6.

Before the group leaves, pass around the basket for prayer partner forms. Have each member draw a form from the basket on his or her way out.

Note: For next week's meeting, invite volunteers to bring in a holiday party food, such as a dip, finger food, or treat, using one of the holiday recipes or one of their own light recipes. If they bring a recipe of their own, ask them to provide copies of the recipe for the other members.

Optional: Have a recipe exchange. Invite members to bring copies of at least one light-eating recipe to share with others.

WEEK FOUR: DO NOT BE AFRAID
Weigh-in and Memory Verse (15 minutes)
Weigh and measure members and listen as they recite the week's Scripture memory verse.

Wellness Spotlight (15 minutes)
In this session, you will experiment with healthy holiday recipes. Read through the "Healthy Holiday Cooking Hints" section in Holiday Sur-

vival Tips, and ask members to share ideas for lightening up their favorite holiday recipes.

Discuss the Christmas menu and recipes and how they plan on utilizing this tool as they plan their Christmas menu.

Optional: Allow time for members to exchange their light holiday recipes while tasting the foods that were brought to the group.

Devotion/Journal Discussion (15 minutes)

Ask members to share with the group how God has shown His love to them this week.

Brainstorm ways that they can show God's love to their neighbors or to the hard-to-love people in their lives.

Prayer Requests/Prayer (15 minutes)

Read Luke 2:9–11. Invite members to pray for strength to face the temptations of the holiday season and they will "not be afraid" (verse 10).

Before the group leaves, pass around the basket for prayer partner forms. Have each member draw a form from the basket on his or her way out.

WEEK FIVE: A NEW CREATION

Weigh-in and Memory Verse (15 minutes)

Weigh and measure members and listen as they recite the week's Scripture memory verse.

Wellness Spotlight (15 minutes)

The holidays can be full of joy, but they can also bring many stresses. It is important your group members learn to manage these negative influences in their lives in order to maintain a healthy and balanced life. Reflecting on this holiday season, ask your group what they can do differently next year to avoid emotional traps.

Have members form pairs and share about holiday stressors. If they feel comfortable, ask them to reflect on any particular days or people that caused them to be especially emotional during the holiday season.

As they review the "Avoid Emotional Traps" section in the Holiday Survival Tips, ask them to plan for next year by evaluating what they could have done differently. Have partners pray for one another.

Devotion/Journal Discussion

Invite members to share about some old things that they need to get rid of this year (attitudes, habits, possessions, and so forth).

Explain that in 2 Corinthians 5:17, Paul suggests that we must "put on" the new self. Invite members to share about how they plan to put on a new self physically, spiritually, emotionally, and mentally.

Have members brainstorm ways that they can support one another to remain faithful to their First Place 4 Health commitment.

Challenge members to bring friends to the next orientation meeting to get the new year off to a great start!

Prayer Requests/Prayer (15 minutes)

Invite members to divide into pairs for a time of prayer. Have each partner pray for the other, asking God to bless them in the coming year and to give them strength to put Him first in their lives.

Before the group leaves, pass around the basket for prayer partner forms. Have each member draw a form from the basket on his or her way out.

WEEK SIX: MAKING A NEW WAY
Weigh-in and Memory Verse (15 minutes)

Weigh and measure members and listen as they recite the week's Scripture memory verse.

Wellness Spotlight (15 minutes)

In this session, the group will focus on spreading joy to others. Before the meeting, gather blank cards and other supplies (construction paper, stickers, felt-tip pens, glue, and so forth) to make greeting cards.

If you have a member who is good with crafts, enlist his or her help in showing members how to make a specific type of card—but keep it simple!

Have each member select one person he or she wants to encourage. Have each member send that person a special New Year's card. Invite volunteers to share about their card's recipient and why they chose that person.

Ask members to plan their New Year's Day menu, using the New Year's Day menu and recipes.

Devotion/Journal Discussion (15 minutes)

Give the members a blank piece of paper and ask them to list anything in their past that they would consider a failure. Have them each silently ask God to forgive them for their part in the failure, and then ask Him to make a way for them to correct the failure and leave the incident in the past.

After a few minutes of private prayer, have members tear up their paper and throw it in the trash (or even have a paper shredder handy for this task). This is a way of putting their failures in the past and forgetting them.

Invite members to share their dreams for the new year by sharing what new thing they would like to accomplish.

Prayer Requests/Prayer (15 minutes)

Invite members to share the areas of commitment or situations in which they need God's power to accomplish a miracle. Pray Isaiah 43:19, asking that God would make a way through their specific situations.

Before the group leaves, pass around the basket for prayer partner forms. Have each member draw a form from the basket on his or her way out.

First Place 4 Health holiday menus & recipes

Each menu plan is based on approximately 1,400 calories. The nutritional information for these meals was calculated using the MasterCook software. It uses a database of over 6,000 food items prepared using United States Department of Agriculture (USDA) publications and information from food manufacturers. As with any nutritional program, MasterCook calculates the nutritional values of the recipes based on ingredients. Nutrition may vary due to how the food is prepared, where the food comes from, soil content, season, ripeners, and processing and methods of preparation. For these reasons, please use the recipes and menu plans as approximate guides. As always, consult your physician and/or registered dietitian before starting a diet program.

For those who need more calories, add the following to the 1,400-calorie plan:

- 1,800 calories: 2 ounce equivalent of meat, 3 ounce equivalent of bread, $1/2$ cup vegetable serving, 1 tsp. fat

- 2,000 calories: 2 ounce equivalent of meat, 4 ounce equivalent of bread, $1/2$ cup vegetable serving, 3 tsp. fat

- 2,200 calories: 2 ounce equivalent of meat, 5 ounce equivalent of bread, $1/2$ cup vegetable serving, $1/2$ cup fruit serving, 5 tsp. fat

- 2,400 calories: 2 ounce equivalent of meat, 6 ounce equivalent of bread, 1 cup vegetable serving, $1/2$ cup fruit serving, 6 tsp. fat

Holiday Grocery List

Produce
- [ ] apples
- [ ] avocado
- [ ] baby arugula
- [ ] bananas
- [ ] basil leaves
- [ ] berries
- [ ] Braeburn apples
- [ ] broccoli
- [ ] Brussels sprouts
- [ ] carrots
- [ ] celery
- [ ] cilantro
- [ ] cranberries
- [ ] garlic, cloves
- [ ] green bell peppers
- [ ] green onions
- [ ] honeydew melon
- [ ] kale
- [ ] kiwifruit
- [ ] lemons
- [ ] limes
- [ ] mangos
- [ ] onions
- [ ] oranges
- [ ] parsnips
- [ ] pineapple
- [ ] plum tomatoes
- [ ] red onion
- [ ] rosemary
- [ ] strawberries
- [ ] sweet potatoes
- [ ] thyme leaves
- [ ] tomatoes
- [ ] zucchini

Baking/Cooking Products
- [ ] baking powder
- [ ] baking soda
- [ ] brown sugar
- [ ] cider vinegar
- [ ] cooking spray
- [ ] egg substitute
- [ ] flour, all-purpose
- [ ] olive oil
- [ ] peppermint extract
- [ ] red food coloring
- [ ] red wine vinegar
- [ ] sugar
- [ ] sugar, brown
- [ ] vanilla extract
- [ ] vegetable shortening
- [ ] yellow cornmeal

Spices
- [ ] black pepper
- [ ] chili powder
- [ ] cinnamon
- [ ] cloves, whole
- [ ] cream of tartar
- [ ] cumin
- [ ] mustard, dry
- [ ] paprika
- [ ] red pepper
- [ ] salt
- [ ] tarragon

Nuts/Seeds
- [ ] pecans
- [ ] pistachios
- [ ] walnuts

Condiments, Spreads and Sauces
- [ ] canola mayonnaise
- [ ] Dijon mustard
- [ ] jelly, all-fruit
- [ ] margarine
- [ ] orange marmalade

- ❏ pesto sauce
- ❏ Ranch dip, low-fat
- ❏ salsa, chunky

Breads, Cereals and Pasta
- ❏ baguette, whole-grain
- ❏ bread, white
- ❏ cornflakes
- ❏ rolled oats, old-fashioned
- ❏ tortillas, whole-wheat

Canned/Frozen Foods
- ❏ apricot halves, dried
- ❏ black beans
- ❏ cream of chicken soup, reduced-fat
- ❏ Great Northern beans
- ❏ hash brown potatoes
- ❏ kidney beans
- ❏ lentils, dry
- ❏ mixed fruit, chunky, in juice
- ❏ refried black beans, fat-free
- ❏ tomato sauce
- ❏ tomatoes, diced
- ❏ vegetable broth

Dairy Products
- ❏ butter
- ❏ buttermilk, low-fat
- ❏ cheddar cheese, low-fat
- ❏ goat cheese
- ❏ Greek yogurt, low-fat
- ❏ Half-and-Half®, fat-free
- ❏ lemon-flavored yogurt, low-fat
- ❏ milk, low-fat
- ❏ sharp cheddar cheese, reduced-fat
- ❏ sour cream, light
- ❏ vanilla yogurt, nonfat
- ❏ whipped topping, light

Juices
- ❏ orange juice

Meat and Poultry
- ❏ beef sirloin steak
- ❏ eggs
- ❏ ground round
- ❏ ham
- ❏ turkey
- ❏ turkey sausage

Thanksgiving Day Menus and Recipes

Note: Recipes for items *italicized in bold* are included below.

MENUS

Breakfast

1 serving ***Overnight Oatmeal with Fruit***

Nutritional Information: 196 calories; 2g fat; 10g protein; 35g carbohydrate; 3g fiber; 3mg cholesterol; 94mg sodium

Thanksgiving Meal

1 (4-oz) serving ***Rosemary-Orange Roast Turkey***
½ cup ***Cheesy Potatoes***
½ cup ***Buttery Brussels Sprouts with Apple***
¼ cup ***Quick and Easy Homemade Cranberry Sauce***
1 serving of ***Apple Pecan Upside-Down Cake***

Nutritional Information: 643 calories; 18g fat; 59g protein; 63g carbohydrate; 8g fiber; 195mg cholesterol; 1073mg sodium

Dinner

1 ***Turkey Tostado***
½ ***Basil and Lime Fruit Salad***

Nutritional Information: 367 calories; 5g fat; 15g protein; 48g carbohydrate; 12g fiber; 24mg cholesterol; 639mg sodium

RECIPES

Overnight Oatmeal with Fruit

¼ cup old-fashioned rolled oats, uncooked
⅓ cup low-fat milk
¼ cup low-fat Greek yogurt
¼ tsp. vanilla extract
1 tbsp. all-fruit jelly
¼ cup of berries (raspberries, strawberries, blueberries, bananas, or blackberries)

In a half pint (1 cup) jar, add oats, milk, yogurt, chia, vanilla, and jelly. Put lid on jar and shake until well combined. Remove lid and add raspberries. Return lid to jar and refrigerate overnight or as long as 2 to 3 days. Eat chilled. Serves 1. (Make-ahead tip: Double or triple—or more!—the recipe to feed family and guests for the holidays.)

Nutrition Information: 196 calories; 2g fat; 10g protein; 35g carbohydrate; 3g fiber; 3mg cholesterol; 94mg sodium

Rosemary-Orange Roast Turkey

Turkey:

- 1 (12-lb.) turkey
- 3 tbsp. rosemary, fresh, finely chopped
- 3 tbsp. orange rind, grated
- 1 tbsp. salt
- 2 tsp. black pepper

Glaze:

- ¼ cup orange marmalade
- ¼ cup orange juice
- 1 tsp. rosemary, fresh, finely chopped
- 1 tbsp. cider vinegar
- 1 tbsp. butter, unsalted
- ¼ tsp. black pepper

To prepare turkey, remove giblets and neck; reserve for another use. Place turkey on a broiler rack on a broiler pan. Starting at neck cavity, loosen skin from breast and drumsticks by inserting fingers, gently pushing between skin and meat. Combine 3 tablespoons rosemary, rind, salt, and 2 teaspoons pepper in a small bowl. Rub rosemary mixture under loosened skin. Tie ends of legs with kitchen string. Lift wing tips up and over back; tuck under turkey. Loosely cover and refrigerate 8 hours (or up to 12 hours). To prepare glaze, combine marmalade, juice, 1 teaspoon rosemary, vinegar, butter, and ¼ teaspoon pepper in a small saucepan; bring to a boil. Reduce heat; simmer 4 minutes or until slightly thickened. Set aside ¼ cup.

Preheat oven to 425° F. Remove turkey from refrigerator and pat dry with a paper towel. Let stand at room temperature 1 hour. Bake at 425° F for 30 minutes or just until the turkey is beginning to brown. Rotate turkey; add 2 cups water to bottom of pan. Reduce oven temperature to 375° F. Cook turkey an additional 60 minutes. Remove turkey from oven; baste with reserved ¼ cup orange mixture. Bake an additional 15 minutes or until thermometer inserted into thickest part of thigh registers 165° F. Remove turkey from oven. Cover loosely with foil and let stand 30 to 60 minutes. Carve turkey; drizzle with remaining ¼ cup orange marmalade mixture. Serves 12.

Nutritional Information: 288 calories; 6g fat; 50g protein; 6g carbohydrate; 1g fiber; 169mg cholesterol; 598mg sodium

Cheesy Potatoes

- 1 (10¾-oz.) can reduced-fat and reduced-sodium condensed cream of chicken soup
- 1 cup (4 oz.) reduced-fat sharp cheddar cheese, shredded
- ½ cup low-fat milk
- ½ cup light sour cream
- ⅓ cup onion, finely chopped, or 2 tbsp. dried minced onion
- ½ tsp. black pepper
- 1 (30-oz.) package shredded or diced hash brown potatoes
- ½ cup cornflakes, crushed, or wheat cereal flakes, crushed

Preheat oven to 350° F. Lightly grease a 2-quart rectangular baking dish; set aside. In a large bowl, combine soup, cheese, milk, sour cream, onion, and pepper. Stir in potatoes. Spread mixture evenly in prepared baking dish. Cover and bake for 45 minutes; stir potatoes. Sprinkle with cornflakes. Bake, uncovered, for 20 to 25 minutes more or until heated through and bubbly. Let stand for 10 minutes before serving. Serves 12.

Nutritional Information: 129 calories; 3g fat; 5g protein; 20g carbohydrate; 1g fiber; 11mg cholesterol; 236mg sodium

Buttery Brussels Sprouts and Apple

- 2 lbs. Brussels sprouts
- ¼ cup butter
- ½ tsp. salt
- 2 tbsp. thyme leaves, fresh
- 2 small Braeburn or other cooking apples, thinly sliced and seeded
- ¼ cup walnuts, toasted and chopped
- ¼ tsp. red pepper, crushed (optional)

Line a 15" x 10" x 1" baking pan with paper towels; set aside. Trim stems and remove any wilted outer leaves from Brussels sprouts. Wash and halve. Bring a large pot of lightly salted water to a boil. Add sprouts and cook, uncovered, for 2 minutes; then drain. Immediately plunge Brussels sprouts into a large bowl of ice water. Let sit for 3 minutes or until cool. Drain well. Transfer to prepared baking pan and pat dry.

Meanwhile, in a 12-inch skillet, melt the butter over medium heat. Cook, stirring often, until the butter begins to brown and smells fragrant and nutty, about 5 to 10 minutes (reduce heat to medium-low, if necessary, to prevent burning). Add the Brussels sprouts and salt. Cook, turning occasionally, for 5 minutes. Add apples and thyme; cook 7 minutes more or until Brussels sprouts are browned and apple is slightly tender, stirring occasionally. Transfer to a serving bowl. Sprinkle with toasted walnuts and crushed red pepper, if desired. Serves 8.

Nutritional Facts: 143 calories; 9g fat; 4g protein; 16g carbohydrate; 5g fiber; 15mg cholesterol; 221mg sodium

Quick and Easy Homemade Cranberry Sauce

1 orange
1 cup sugar
¼ cup water
1 (12-oz.) package fresh cranberries

Grate orange to yield 2 teaspoons rind. Cut orange in half; squeeze to yield ½ cup juice. Combine rind, juice, sugar, water, and cranberries in a small saucepan; bring to a boil. Reduce heat to low and simmer 7 minutes or until cranberries begin to pop. Remove from heat; cover and refrigerate at least 30 minutes. Serves 12.

Nutritional Information: 83 calories; 0g fat; 0g protein; 21g carbohydrate; 1g fiber; 0mg cholesterol; 1mg sodium

Apple-Pecan Upside-Down Cake

¼ cup butter
½ cup eggs
cooking spray
1 cup flour, all-purpose
2 tsp. cinnamon, ground
1 tsp. baking powder
¼ tsp. salt
½ cup sugar, brown (packed)
¼ cup sugar, granulated
1 tsp. vanilla extract
½ cup pecans, toasted and coarsely
  ground
½ tsp. lemon peel, finely shredded
3 cups apples (such as Jonathan, Rome,
  or Golden Delicious), sliced
whipped topping, light (optional)

Let butter and eggs stand at room temperature for 30 minutes. Meanwhile, line a 9" x 9" x 2" baking pan with foil. Coat foil with cooking spray; set aside. In a small bowl, stir together flour, cinnamon, baking powder, and salt; set aside. Preheat oven to 350° F. In a medium bowl, beat butter with an electric mixer on medium to high speed for 30 seconds. Add brown sugar and granulated sugar, beating on medium speed until combined and scraping bowl as needed. Beat on medium speed for 2 minutes more. Beat in egg and vanilla. Add flour mixture; beat until combined. Stir in pecans and lemon peel. Arrange the 3 cups apple slices in the prepared pan. Spread the pecan mixture over apples (the batter will be thick). Bake 25 to 30 minutes or until a toothpick inserted near the center comes out clean. Cool cake in pan on a wire rack for 5 minutes. Invert cake onto a platter. Carefully remove the foil. Serve warm (cut the cake into squares to serve). If desired, top each serving low-fat dessert topping. Serves 12.

Nutritional Information: 176 calories; 7g fat; 3g protein; 26g carbohydrate; 2g fiber; 11mg cholesterol; 121mg sodium

Turkey Tostadas

4 (8-inch) whole-wheat tortillas
cooking spray
1 (16-oz.) can fat-free refried black beans
¾ cup bottled chunky salsa, divided
1½ cups cooked turkey, shredded
1 cup (4 oz.) sharp cheddar cheese, low-fat, shredded
1 cup tomato, chopped
½ avocado, peeled and cut into 12 slices
¼ cup cilantro, fresh, chopped

Preheat oven to 425° F. Spray both sides of each tortilla with cooking spray; arrange on large baking sheet. Bake at 425° F for 3½ minutes on each side or until lightly toasted. Combine beans and ¼ cup salsa in a microwave-safe bowl; cover with plastic wrap. Microwave on high for 4 minutes or until thoroughly heated, stirring after 2 minutes; set aside. Combine turkey and ½ cup salsa in a microwave-safe bowl; cover with plastic wrap. Microwave on high for 2 minutes or until thoroughly heated. Divide bean mixture among tortillas; top with turkey mixture. Sprinkle with cheese; top with tomato. Arrange 3 avocado slices over each tostada; sprinkle each evenly with cilantro. Serves 4.

Nutritional Information: 275 calories; 5g fat; 14g protein; 25g carbohydrate; 10g fiber; 24mg cholesterol; 619mg sodium

Basil and Lime Fruit Salad

½ cup sugar
½ cup water
½ cup basil leaves, packed
1 tbsp. lime rind, grated
4 cups pineapple, cubed
3 cups strawberries, quartered
2 cups mango, cubed and peeled
4 kiwifruit, peeled, halved lengthwise, and sliced

Combine sugar and ½ cup water in a saucepan; bring to a boil. Cook 1 minute or until sugar dissolves. Remove from heat; stir in basil and rind. Cool. Strain sugar mixture into a bowl; discard solids. Combine pineapple and remaining ingredients in a large bowl. Drizzle with sugar mixture; toss gently. Serves 12.

Nutrition Information: 92 calories; 0g fat; 1g protein; 24g carbohydrate; 2g fiber; 0mg cholesterol; 2mg sodium

Christmas Day Menus and Recipes

Note: Recipes for items *italicized in bold* are included below.

MENUS

Breakfast
1 serving of cubed peeled ½ cup *Easy Fruit Salad*

Nutritional Information: 283 calories; 7g fat; 17g protein; 39g carbohydrate; 3g fiber; 76mg cholesterol; 660mg sodium

Christmas Meal
4 oz. *Glazed Ham with Apricots* ½ cup *Broccoli with Dijon*
½ cup *Mashed Sweet Potatoes with* *Vinaigrette*
   Goat Cheese 1 serving of *Apple Cranberry Crisp*

Nutritional Information: 620 calories; 14g fat; 30g protein; 74g carbohydrate; 10g fiber; 79mg cholesterol; 2047mg sodium

Dinner
1 serving of *Crockpot Vegetable Soup* 2 *Meringue Cookies*
1 *Green Onion Biscuit*

Nutritional Information: 274 calories; 6g fat; 12g protein; 11g carbohydrate; 5g fiber; 23mg cholesterol; 153mg sodium

RECIPES

Sausage and Cheese Breakfast Casserole

12 oz. turkey sausage
2 cups low-fat milk
2 cups egg substitute
1 tsp. dry mustard
¾ tsp. salt
½ tsp. black pepper
¼ tsp. red pepper
3 large eggs
16 (1 oz.) slices white bread
1 cup (4 oz.) reduced-fat extra sharp
   cheddar cheese, finely shredded
¼ tsp. paprika
cooking spray

Heat a large nonstick skillet over medium-high heat. Coat pan with cooking spray. Add sausage to pan and cook for 5 minutes or until browned, stirring and breaking sausage to crumble. Remove from heat and cool. Combine milk, egg substitute, mustard, salt, black pepper, red pepper and eggs in a large bowl, stirring with a whisk. Trim crusts from bread. Cut bread into 1-inch cubes and add bread cubes, sausage and cheddar cheese to milk mixture, stirring to combine. Pour bread mixture into a 13" x 9" baking dish or a three-quart casserole dish coated with cooking spray. Spread egg mixture evenly in baking dish. Cover and refrigerate 8 hours or overnight. Preheat oven to 350° F. Remove casserole from refrigerator and let stand for 30 minutes. Sprinkle paprika evenly over the casserole. Bake at 350° F for 45 minutes or until set and lightly browned. Let stand for 10 minutes. Serves 12.

Nutritional Information: 184 calories; 7g fat 16g protein; 14g carbohydrate; 1g fiber; 76mg cholesterol; 636mg sodium

Easy Fruit Salad

2 tbsp. sugar
1 tsp. orange rind, grated
2 tbsp. orange juice
3 cups honeydew melon, cubed
1 cup strawberries, sliced
1 kiwifruit, sliced and peeled

Place sugar, orange rind and orange juice in a large bowl; stir until sugar dissolves. Add honeydew, strawberries, and kiwifruit; toss gently to combine. Serves 4.

Nutrition Information: 99 calories; 0g fat; 1g protein; 25g carbohydrate; 3g fiber; 0mg cholesterol; 24mg sodium

Glazed Ham with Apricots

1 bone-in smoked half ham, fully cooked
1 package dried apricot halves
2 tbsp. whole cloves
½ cup orange marmalade or apricot jam
2 tbsp. country-style Dijon mustard with seeds

Preheat oven to 325° F. With a knife, remove skin and trim all but $1/8$ inch fat from ham. Secure apricots with cloves to fat side of ham in rows, leaving some space between apricots. Place ham, fat side up, on rack in large roasting pan (17" x 11½"); add 1 cup water. Cover pan tightly with foil. Bake 2 hours. After ham has baked 1 hour and 45 minutes, prepare glaze. In a 1-quart saucepan, heat marmalade and mustard to boiling on medium-high. Remove foil from ham and carefully brush with some glaze. Continue to bake ham 30 to 40 minutes longer or until meat thermometer reaches 135° F, brushing with glaze every 15 minutes. Internal temperature of ham will rise 5° to 10° F on standing. (Some apricots may fall off into pan as you glaze.) Transfer ham to cutting board; cover and let stand 20 minutes for easier slicing. Slice ham and serve with apricots from pan. Serves 16.

Nutritional Information: 209 calories; 2g fat; 20g protein; 2g carbohydrate; 0g fiber; 67mg cholesterol; 1505mg sodium.

Mashed Sweet Potatoes with Goat Cheese

3 lbs. sweet potatoes, peeled and cubed
½ cup pistachios, chopped
¼ cup fat-free Half-and-Half®

2 tbsp. plus 1 tsp. butter, divided
2 oz. goat cheese

Place potatoes in 3-quart saucepan with enough water to cover. Season with a little salt and pepper. Bring to a boil and reduce heat to a simmer for about 10 minutes. While potatoes are cooking, melt 1 teaspoon butter in saucepan and add about ½ cup of chopped pistachio. Toss and cook over medium heat for 1 to 2 minutes until toasted. Set aside. When potatoes are tender, drain and return to saucepan. Melt 2 tablespoons butter and add to potatoes with Half-and-Half. Mash potatoes to desired consistency and stir in goat cheese. When ready to serve sprinkle with toasted pistachios. Serves 12.

Nutritional Information: 146 calories; 5g fat; 3g protein; 21g carbohydrate; 3g fiber; 11mg cholesterol; 55mg sodium

Broccoli with Dijon Vinaigrette

2¼ lbs. broccoli, fresh
2 tsp. olive oil
¼ cup green onions, finely chopped
½ tsp. dried tarragon
½ tsp. dry mustard
3 cloves garlic, minced

2 tbsp. red wine vinegar
2 tbsp. water
1 tbsp. Dijon mustard
⅛ tsp. salt
¼ tsp. black pepper

Remove broccoli leaves and cut off tough ends of stalks; discard. Wash broccoli and cut into spears. Arrange broccoli in a steamer basket over boiling water. Cover and steam 6 minutes or until crisp-tender. Place in a serving bowl; keep warm. Heat oil in a small saucepan over medium heat. Add green onions, tarragon, mustard, and garlic; sauté for 3 minutes. Remove from heat; add vinegar and remaining 4 ingredients, stirring with a wire whisk until blended. Drizzle over broccoli, tossing gently to coat. Serves 8.

Nutritional Information: 52 calories; 2g fat; 4g protein; 8g carbohydrate; 4g fiber; 0mg cholesterol; 126mg sodium

Apple Cranberry Crisp

5 cups apples, thinly sliced and peeled
1 cup cranberries
2 tbsp. sugar
½ cup old-fashioned rolled oats
⅓ cup brown sugar, packed
3 tbsp. all-purpose flour
½ tsp. ground cinnamon
2 tbsp. margarine
½ cup vanilla or lemon nonfat yogurt

In a large mixing bowl combine apples, cranberries, and granulated sugar. Transfer to a 2-quart square baking dish or a 9-inch pie plate. In a small bowl combine oats, brown sugar, flour, and cinnamon. Cut in margarine until crumbly. Sprinkle oat mixture evenly over apple mixture. Bake in a 375° F oven for 30 to 35 minutes or until apples are tender. Serve warm with a dollop of vanilla or lemon yogurt. Serves 6.

Nutritional Information: 213 calories; 5g fat; 3g protein; 43g carbohydrate; 3g fiber; 1mg cholesterol; 61mg sodium

Healthy Crockpot Vegetable Soup

1 cup onions, chopped
1 cup carrots, sliced
1 cup zucchini, sliced
1 cup dry lentils
1 cup parsnips, chopped
1 cup celery, diced
1 cup turkey sausage
4 cups vegetable broth
salt
black pepper
2 cups chopped kale

Put all ingredients but kale in crockpot on low for six or more hours. Add kale 5 minutes before serving and cook until wilted. Serves 8. (Tip: If you don't have a lot of time or a crockpot, you can cook in a large saucepan. Bring all ingredients to a boil and then lower to a simmer for one hour.)

Nutritional Information: 150 calories; 3g fat; 10g protein; 21g carbohydrate; 4g fiber; 2mg cholesterol; 184mg sodium

Green Onion Biscuits

2 cups all-purpose flour
2 tsp. baking powder
½ tsp. salt
¼ tsp. baking soda

3 tbsp. vegetable shortening
¼ cup green onions, finely chopped
1 cup low-fat buttermilk
cooking spray

Preheat oven to 400° F. Combine flour, baking powder, salt, and baking soda in a large bowl; cut in shortening with a pastry blender or 2 knives until mixture resembles coarse meal. Stir in green onions. Add buttermilk, stirring just until flour mixture is moist. Drop batter by heaping tablespoons onto a baking sheet coated with cooking spray. Bake at 400° F for 15 minutes or until lightly browned. Makes 16 biscuits.

Nutritional Information: 97 calories; 3g fat; 2g protein; 16g carbohydrate; 1g fiber; 21mg cholesterol; 48mg sodium

Holiday Meringues

3 egg whites
¼ tsp. cream of tartar
⅛ tsp. salt

¾ cup sugar
⅛ tsp. peppermint extract
red food coloring

Preheat oven to 200° F. Line a cookie sheet with parchment paper; set aside. In a large mixing bowl beat egg whites, cream of tartar, and salt with an electric mixer on medium speed until soft peaks form (tips curl). Gradually add sugar, about ½ tablespoon at a time, beating on high speed until stiff peaks form (tips stand straight). Fold in extract and two drops of food coloring (mixture may soften slightly). Spoon egg white mixture in 2-inch dollops, 1 inch apart onto the prepared cookie sheet. Bake about 1½ hours or until meringues appear dry and are firm when lightly touched. Transfer cookies to a wire rack; cool. Makes 36 cookies. (Note: Instead of peppermint extract and food coloring, you can also add ¼ cup of mini chocolate chips to make a *Chocolate Chip Meringue*.)

To store: Layer cookies between sheets of waxed paper in an airtight container; cover. Store at room temperature for up to 3 days or freeze for up to 3 months.

Nutritional Information: 27 calories; 0g fat; 0g protein; 6g carbohydrate; 0g fiber; 0mg cholesterol; 20mg sodium

New Year's Day Menus and Recipes

Note: Recipes for items *italicized in bold* are included below.

MENUS

Breakfast
2 servings of *Eggs in Hash Brown Nests*

1 cup of fruit (your choice—sliced strawberries, blueberries, apples, etc.)

Nutritional Information: 192 calories; 6g fat; 8g protein; 28g carbohydrate; 6g fiber; 212mg cholesterol; 80mg sodium

New Year's Day Meal
1 serving of *Chili con Carne*
1 serving of *Blue Ribbon Cornbread*

1 serving of *Creamy Fruit Salad*

Nutritional Information: 743 calories; 9g fat; 33g protein; 142g carbohydrate; 24g fiber; 22mg cholesterol; 1602mg sodium

Dinner
1 *Steak Baguette with Pesto Mayo*

1 cup carrot sticks with low-fat Ranch dip

Nutritional Information: 391 calories; 9g fat; 21g protein; 41g carbohydrate; 5g fiber; 26mg cholesterol; 701mg sodium

RECIPES

Eggs in Hash Brown Nests
1 medium sweet potato, washed and peeled

4 large eggs

Preheat oven to 400°F and grease 4 cups in a regular-size muffin tin with coconut oil. Using a coarse cheese grater, grate the sweet potato into a medium-size bowl. Using your fingers, line the 4 greased muffin tins with the sweet potatoes, pressing the sweet potatoes up against the sides to make a "crust." Bake the sweet potato crusts for 5 to 8 minutes, making sure not to burn the sweet potatoes. Remove the muffin tin from the oven and carefully crack an egg in each mini-crust. Place the muffin tin back in the oven and bake for 15 to 20 minutes or until the egg whites are opaque. Allow the egg nests to cool before removing from the muffin tin. Serves 2 (two *Egg Nests* each).

Nutritional Information: 142 calories; 6g fat; 8g protein; 16g carbohydrate; 2g fiber; 212mg cholesterol; 78mg sodium

Chili con Carne

2 lbs. ground round
1 (15-oz.) can kidney beans
1 (15-oz.) can black beans
1 (15-oz.) can Great Northern beans
2 (16-oz.) cans diced tomatoes
2 large onions, chopped
2 (8-oz.) cans tomato sauce
2 green bell peppers, chopped
¼ tsp. paprika
2 tbsp. chili powder
2 tsp. ground cumin

In large pot, cook ground beef until fully browned. Add rest of ingredients and stir to blend well. Bring to a boil; cover and simmer for 1 hour. Serves 8. (Note: For a vegetarian alternative, use two 12-oz. packages ground beef substitute.)

Nutritional Information: 524 calories; 7g fat; 27g protein; 95g carbohydrate; 20g fiber; 0mg cholesterol; 1304mg sodium

Blue Ribbon Cornbread

1 cup yellow cornmeal
1 cup flour, all-purpose
½ tsp. salt
1 tbsp. baking powder
1 egg
1 cup low-fat milk
4 oz. nonfat vanilla yogurt, sugar-free
cooking spray

Sift together dry ingredients in bowl. Add egg, milk, and yogurt; beat together one minute. Spray a 9" x 9" or 9" x 13" baking dish with cooking spray and pour in mixture. Bake at 425° F for 20 minutes. Serves 10.

Variations:
- Replace yogurt with 1-cup cream-style corn
- Replace milk with 1-cup buttermilk (made from skim milk)

Nutritional Information: 118 calories; 1g fat; 4g protein; 23g carbohydrate; 1g fiber; 22mg cholesterol; 280mg sodium

Creamy Fruit Salad

1 (15-oz.) can chunky mixed fruit in juice, drained
2 medium bananas, sliced
1 cup strawberries, sliced
½ cup lemon-flavored low-fat yogurt, sugar-free
½ cup whipped topping, light

Combine mixed fruit, bananas, and strawberries in medium bowl. Gently fold in yogurt and whipped topping until fruit is coated. Refrigerate until ready to serve. Serves 4.

Nutritional Information: 101 calories; 1g fat; 2g protein; 24g carbohydrate; 3g fiber; 0mg cholesterol; 18mg sodium

Steak Baguettes with Pesto Mayo

1 (12-oz.) boneless beef sirloin steak (about 1 inch thick), trimmed
⅛ tsp. black pepper
2 tbsp. canola mayonnaise
2 tbsp. pesto sauce, refrigerated
1 (12-oz.) piece white or whole-grain baguette, split in half horizontally
¼ tsp. salt
1 cup baby arugula, packed (about 1 oz.)
3 (⅛-inch-thick) red onion slices
2 plum tomatoes, thinly sliced lengthwise

Heat a grill pan over medium-high heat. Sprinkle steak with salt and pepper. Add steak to pan and cook 2½ minutes on each side or until desired degree of doneness. Remove the steak from pan and let stand for 5 minutes. Cut steak across grain into thin slices. Combine mayonnaise and pesto, stirring until well blended. Spread mayonnaise mixture evenly over cut sides of bread. Layer bottom half of bread with arugula, red onion, steak, and tomato; top with top half of bread. Cut sandwich diagonally into 4 equal pieces. Serves 4.

Nutritional Information: 346 calories; 9g fat; 21g protein; 41g carbohydrate; 2g fiber; 26mg cholesterol; 701mg sodium

Member Survey

Please answer the following questions to help your leader plan your First Place 4 Health meetings so that your needs might be met in this session. Give this form to your leader at the first group meeting.

Name _____   Birth date _____

Please list those who live in your household.

Name	Relationship	Age

What church do you attend? _____

Are you interested in receiving more information about our church?

    Yes   No

Occupation _____

What talent or area of expertise would you be willing to share with our class?

_____

Why did you join First Place 4 Health?

_____

With notice, would you be willing to lead a Bible study discussion one week?

    Yes   No

Are you comfortable praying out loud? _____

If the assistant leader were absent, would you be willing to assist in weighing in members and possibly evaluating the Live It Trackers?

    Yes   No

Any other comments:

_____
_____

Personal Weight and Measurement Record

Week	Weight	+ or -	Goal this Session	Pounds to goal
1				
2				
3				
4				
5				
6				
7				
8				
9				
10				
11				
12				

Beginning Measurements

Waist _____ Hips _____ Thighs _____ Chest _____

Ending Measurements

Waist _____ Hips _____ Thighs _____ Chest _____

First Place 4 Health
Prayer Partner

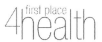

A JOY-FULL
SEASON
Week 1

Now, our God, we give you thanks, and praise your glorious name.
1 CHRONICLES 29:13

Date: _____

Name: _____

Home Phone: (___) _____

Work Phone: (___) _____

Email: _____

Personal Prayer Concerns:

_____

_____

_____

_____

_____

_____

This form is for prayer requests that are personal to you and your journey in First Place 4 Health. Please complete this form and have it ready to turn in when you arrive at your group meeting.

First Place 4 Health
Prayer Partner

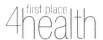

A JOY-FULL SEASON
Week 2

I will give you thanks, for you answered me; you have become my salvation.
PSALM 118:21

Date: _____

Name: _____

Home Phone: (____) _____

Work Phone: (____) _____

Email: _____

Personal Prayer Concerns:

_____

_____

_____

_____

_____

_____

This form is for prayer requests that are personal to you and your journey in First Place 4 Health. Please complete this form and have it ready to turn in when you arrive at your group meeting.

First Place 4 Health
Prayer Partner

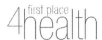

A JOY-FULL SEASON
Week 3

For to us a child is born, to us a son is given, and the government will be on his shoulders. And he will be called Wonderful Counselor, Mighty God, Everlasting Father, Prince of Peace.
ISAIAH 9:6

Date:

Name:

Home Phone: (   )

Work Phone: (   )

Email:

Personal Prayer Concerns:

This form is for prayer requests that are personal to you and your journey in First Place 4 Health. Please complete this form and have it ready to turn in when you arrive at your group meeting.

First Place 4 Health
Prayer Partner

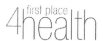

A JOY-FULL SEASON
Week 4

An angel of the Lord appeared to them, and the glory of the Lord shone around them, and they were terrified. But the angel said to them, "Do not be afraid. I bring you good news that will cause great joy for all the people. Today in the town of David a Savior has been born to you; he is the Messiah, the Lord.

Date: _____

Name: _____

Home Phone: (___) _____

Work Phone: (___) _____

Email: _____

Personal Prayer Concerns:

_____
_____
_____
_____
_____
_____
_____

This form is for prayer requests that are personal to you and your journey in First Place 4 Health. Please complete this form and have it ready to turn in when you arrive at your group meeting.

First Place 4 Health
Prayer Partner

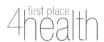

A JOY-FULL SEASON
Week 5

*Therefore, if anyone is in Christ, the new creation has come:
The old has gone, the new is here!*
2 CORINTHIANS 5:17

Date: _____

Name: _____

Home Phone: (____) _____

Work Phone: (____) _____

Email: _____

Personal Prayer Concerns:

_____

_____

_____

_____

_____

_____

_____

This form is for prayer requests that are personal to you and your journey in First Place 4 Health. Please complete this form and have it ready to turn in when you arrive at your group meeting.

First Place 4 Health
Prayer Partner

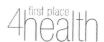

A JOY-FULL SEASON
Week 6

*See, I am doing a new thing! Now it springs up; do you not perceive it?
I am making a way in the wilderness and streams in the wasteland.*
ISAIAH 43:19

Date: _____

Name: _____

Home Phone: (___) _____

Work Phone: (___) _____

Email: _____

Personal Prayer Concerns:

_____
_____
_____
_____
_____
_____

This form is for prayer requests that are personal to you and your journey in First Place 4 Health. Please complete this form and have it ready to turn in when you arrive at your group meeting.

Live It Tracker

Name: _____ Loss/gain: _____ lbs.
Date: _____ Week #: ____ Calorie Range: _____ My food goal for next week: _____
Activity Level: None, < 30 min/day, 30-60 min/day, 60+ min/day   My activity goal for next week: _____

Group	Daily Calories							
	1300-1400	1500-1600	1700-1800	1900-2000	2100-2200	2300-2400	2500-2600	2700-2800
Fruits	1.5-2 c.	1.5-2 c.	1.5-2 c.	2-2.5 c.	2-2.5 c.	2.5-3.5 c.	3.5-4.5 c.	3.5-4.5 c.
Vegetables	1.5-2 c.	2-2.5 c.	2.5-3 c.	2.5-3 c.	3-3.5 c.	3.5-4.5 c.	4.5-5 c.	4.5-5 c.
Grains	5 oz-eq.	5-6 oz-eq.	6-7 oz-eq.	6-7 oz-eq.	7-8 oz-eq.	8-9 oz-eq.	9-10 oz-eq.	10-11 oz-eq.
Meat & Beans	4 oz-eq.	5 oz-eq.	5-5.5 oz-eq.	5.5-6.5 oz-eq.	6.5-7 oz-eq.	7-7.5 oz-eq.	7-7.5 oz-eq.	7.5-8 oz-eq.
Milk	2-3 c.	3 c.	3 c.	3 c.	3 c.	3 c.	3 c.	3 c.
Healthy Oils	4 tsp.	5 tsp.	5 tsp.	6 tsp.	6 tsp.	7 tsp.	8 tsp.	8 tsp.

Day/Date: _____

Breakfast: _____ Lunch: _____

Dinner: _____ Snack: _____

Group	Fruits	Vegetables	Grains	Meat & Beans	Milk	Oils
Goal Amount						
Estimate Your Total						
Increase ⇧ or Decrease? ⇩						

Physical Activity: _____ Spiritual Activity: _____
Steps/Miles/Minutes: _____

Day/Date: _____

Breakfast: _____ Lunch: _____

Dinner: _____ Snack: _____

Group	Fruits	Vegetables	Grains	Meat & Beans	Milk	Oils
Goal Amount						
Estimate Your Total						
Increase ⇧ or Decrease? ⇩						

Physical Activity: _____ Spiritual Activity: _____
Steps/Miles/Minutes: _____

Day/Date: _____

Breakfast: _____ Lunch: _____

Dinner: _____ Snack: _____

Group	Fruits	Vegetables	Grains	Meat & Beans	Milk	Oils
Goal Amount						
Estimate Your Total						
Increase ⇧ or Decrease? ⇩						

Physical Activity: _____ Spiritual Activity: _____
Steps/Miles/Minutes: _____

Day/Date: _____

Breakfast: _____ Lunch: _____

Dinner: _____ Snack: _____

Group	Fruits	Vegetables	Grains	Meat & Beans	Milk	Oils
Goal Amount						
Estimate Your Total						
Increase ⇧ or Decrease? ⇩						

Physical Activity: _____ Spiritual Activity: _____

Steps/Miles/Minutes: _____

Day/Date: _____

Breakfast: _____ Lunch: _____

Dinner: _____ Snack: _____

Group	Fruits	Vegetables	Grains	Meat & Beans	Milk	Oils
Goal Amount						
Estimate Your Total						
Increase ⇧ or Decrease? ⇩						

Physical Activity: _____ Spiritual Activity: _____

Steps/Miles/Minutes: _____

Day/Date: _____

Breakfast: _____ Lunch: _____

Dinner: _____ Snack: _____

Group	Fruits	Vegetables	Grains	Meat & Beans	Milk	Oils
Goal Amount						
Estimate Your Total						
Increase ⇧ or Decrease? ⇩						

Physical Activity: _____ Spiritual Activity: _____

Steps/Miles/Minutes: _____

Day/Date: _____

Breakfast: _____ Lunch: _____

Dinner: _____ Snack: _____

Group	Fruits	Vegetables	Grains	Meat & Beans	Milk	Oils
Goal Amount						
Estimate Your Total						
Increase ⇧ or Decrease? ⇩						

Physical Activity: _____ Spiritual Activity: _____

Steps/Miles/Minutes: _____

Copyright 2009 First Place 4 Health. Do not duplicate without permission from First Place 4 Health.

Live It Tracker

Name: _____ Loss/gain: _____ lbs.

Date: _____ Week #: _____ Calorie Range: _____ My food goal for next week: _____

Activity Level: None, < 30 min/day, 30-60 min/day, 60+ min/day   My activity goal for next week: _____

Group	Daily Calories							
	1300-1400	1500-1600	1700-1800	1900-2000	2100-2200	2300-2400	2500-2600	2700-2800
Fruits	1.5-2 c.	1.5-2 c.	1.5-2 c.	2-2.5 c.	2-2.5 c.	2.5-3.5 c.	3.5-4.5 c.	3.5-4.5 c.
Vegetables	1.5-2 c.	2-2.5 c.	2.5-3 c.	2.5-3 c.	3-3.5 c.	3.5-4.5 c.	4.5-5 c.	4.5-5 c.
Grains	5 oz-eq.	5-6 oz-eq.	6-7 oz-eq.	6-7 oz-eq.	7-8 oz-eq.	8-9 oz-eq.	9-10 oz-eq.	10-11 oz-eq.
Meat & Beans	4 oz-eq.	5 oz-eq.	5-5.5 oz-eq.	5.5-6.5 oz-eq.	6.5-7 oz-eq.	7-7.5 oz-eq.	7-7.5 oz-eq.	7.5-8 oz-eq.
Milk	2-3 c.	3 c.	3 c.	3 c.	3 c.	3 c.	3 c.	3 c.
Healthy Oils	4 tsp.	5 tsp.	5 tsp.	6 tsp.	6 tsp.	7 tsp.	8 tsp.	8 tsp.

Day/Date: _____

Breakfast: _____ Lunch: _____

Dinner: _____ Snack: _____

Group	Fruits	Vegetables	Grains	Meat & Beans	Milk	Oils
Goal Amount						
Estimate Your Total						
Increase ⇧ or Decrease? ⇩						

Physical Activity: _____ Spiritual Activity: _____

Steps/Miles/Minutes: _____

Day/Date: _____

Breakfast: _____ Lunch: _____

Dinner: _____ Snack: _____

Group	Fruits	Vegetables	Grains	Meat & Beans	Milk	Oils
Goal Amount						
Estimate Your Total						
Increase ⇧ or Decrease? ⇩						

Physical Activity: _____ Spiritual Activity: _____

Steps/Miles/Minutes: _____

Day/Date: _____

Breakfast: _____ Lunch: _____

Dinner: _____ Snack: _____

Group	Fruits	Vegetables	Grains	Meat & Beans	Milk	Oils
Goal Amount						
Estimate Your Total						
Increase ⇧ or Decrease? ⇩						

Physical Activity: _____ Spiritual Activity: _____

Steps/Miles/Minutes: _____

Copyright 2009 First Place 4 Health. Do not duplicate without permission from First Place 4 Health.

Day/Date:

Breakfast: _____ Lunch: _____

Dinner: _____ Snack: _____

Group	Fruits	Vegetables	Grains	Meat & Beans	Milk	Oils
Goal Amount						
Estimate Your Total						
Increase ⇧ or Decrease? ⇩						

Physical Activity: _____ Spiritual Activity: _____

Steps/Miles/Minutes: _____

Day/Date:

Breakfast: _____ Lunch: _____

Dinner: _____ Snack: _____

Group	Fruits	Vegetables	Grains	Meat & Beans	Milk	Oils
Goal Amount						
Estimate Your Total						
Increase ⇧ or Decrease? ⇩						

Physical Activity: _____ Spiritual Activity: _____

Steps/Miles/Minutes: _____

Day/Date:

Breakfast: _____ Lunch: _____

Dinner: _____ Snack: _____

Group	Fruits	Vegetables	Grains	Meat & Beans	Milk	Oils
Goal Amount						
Estimate Your Total						
Increase ⇧ or Decrease? ⇩						

Physical Activity: _____ Spiritual Activity: _____

Steps/Miles/Minutes: _____

Day/Date:

Breakfast: _____ Lunch: _____

Dinner: _____ Snack: _____

Group	Fruits	Vegetables	Grains	Meat & Beans	Milk	Oils
Goal Amount						
Estimate Your Total						
Increase ⇧ or Decrease? ⇩						

Physical Activity: _____ Spiritual Activity: _____

Steps/Miles/Minutes: _____

Live It Tracker

Name: _____ Loss/gain: _____ lbs.

Date: _____ Week #: ____ Calorie Range: _____ My food goal for next week: _____

Activity Level: None, < 30 min/day, 30-60 min/day, 60+ min/day   My activity goal for next week: _____

Group	Daily Calories							
	1300-1400	1500-1600	1700-1800	1900-2000	2100-2200	2300-2400	2500-2600	2700-2800
Fruits	1.5-2 c.	1.5-2 c.	1.5-2 c.	2-2.5 c.	2-2.5 c.	2.5-3.5 c.	3.5-4.5 c.	3.5-4.5 c.
Vegetables	1.5-2 c.	2-2.5 c.	2.5-3 c.	2.5-3 c.	3-3.5 c.	3.5-4.5 c.	4.5-5 c.	4.5-5 c.
Grains	5 oz-eq.	5-6 oz-eq.	6-7 oz-eq.	6-7 oz-eq.	7-8 oz-eq.	8-9 oz-eq.	9-10 oz-eq.	10-11 oz-eq.
Meat & Beans	4 oz-eq.	5 oz-eq.	5-5.5 oz-eq.	5.5-6.5 oz-eq.	6.5-7 oz-eq.	7-7.5 oz-eq.	7-7.5 oz-eq.	7.5-8 oz-eq.
Milk	2-3 c.	3 c.	3 c.	3 c.	3 c.	3 c.	3 c.	3 c.
Healthy Oils	4 tsp.	5 tsp.	5 tsp.	6 tsp.	6 tsp.	7 tsp.	8 tsp.	8 tsp.

Day/Date: _____

Breakfast: _____   Lunch: _____

Dinner: _____   Snack: _____

Group	Fruits	Vegetables	Grains	Meat & Beans	Milk	Oils
Goal Amount						
Estimate Your Total						
Increase ⇧ or Decrease? ⇩						

Physical Activity: _____   Spiritual Activity: _____

Steps/Miles/Minutes: _____

Day/Date: _____

Breakfast: _____   Lunch: _____

Dinner: _____   Snack: _____

Group	Fruits	Vegetables	Grains	Meat & Beans	Milk	Oils
Goal Amount						
Estimate Your Total						
Increase ⇧ or Decrease? ⇩						

Physical Activity: _____   Spiritual Activity: _____

Steps/Miles/Minutes: _____

Day/Date: _____

Breakfast: _____   Lunch: _____

Dinner: _____   Snack: _____

Group	Fruits	Vegetables	Grains	Meat & Beans	Milk	Oils
Goal Amount						
Estimate Your Total						
Increase ⇧ or Decrease? ⇩						

Physical Activity: _____   Spiritual Activity: _____

Steps/Miles/Minutes: _____

Day/Date: _____

Breakfast: _____ Lunch: _____

Dinner: _____ Snack: _____

Group	Fruits	Vegetables	Grains	Meat & Beans	Milk	Oils
Goal Amount						
Estimate Your Total						
Increase ⇧ or Decrease? ⇩						

Physical Activity: _____ Spiritual Activity: _____

Steps/Miles/Minutes: _____

Day/Date: _____

Breakfast: _____ Lunch: _____

Dinner: _____ Snack: _____

Group	Fruits	Vegetables	Grains	Meat & Beans	Milk	Oils
Goal Amount						
Estimate Your Total						
Increase ⇧ or Decrease? ⇩						

Physical Activity: _____ Spiritual Activity: _____

Steps/Miles/Minutes: _____

Day/Date: _____

Breakfast: _____ Lunch: _____

Dinner: _____ Snack: _____

Group	Fruits	Vegetables	Grains	Meat & Beans	Milk	Oils
Goal Amount						
Estimate Your Total						
Increase ⇧ or Decrease? ⇩						

Physical Activity: _____ Spiritual Activity: _____

Steps/Miles/Minutes: _____

Day/Date: _____

Breakfast: _____ Lunch: _____

Dinner: _____ Snack: _____

Group	Fruits	Vegetables	Grains	Meat & Beans	Milk	Oils
Goal Amount						
Estimate Your Total						
Increase ⇧ or Decrease? ⇩						

Physical Activity: _____ Spiritual Activity: _____

Steps/Miles/Minutes: _____

Live It Tracker

Name: _____ Loss/gain: _____ lbs.

Date: _____ Week #: ____ Calorie Range: _____ My food goal for next week: _____

Activity Level: None, < 30 min/day, 30-60 min/day, 60+ min/day   My activity goal for next week: _____

Group	Daily Calories							
	1300-1400	1500-1600	1700-1800	1900-2000	2100-2200	2300-2400	2500-2600	2700-2800
Fruits	1.5-2 c.	1.5-2 c.	1.5-2 c.	2-2.5 c.	2-2.5 c.	2.5-3.5 c.	3.5-4.5 c.	3.5-4.5 c.
Vegetables	1.5-2 c.	2-2.5 c.	2.5-3 c.	2.5-3 c.	3-3.5 c.	3.5-4.5 c.	4.5-5 c.	4.5-5 c.
Grains	5 oz-eq.	5-6 oz-eq.	6-7 oz-eq.	6-7 oz-eq.	7-8 oz-eq.	8-9 oz-eq.	9-10 oz-eq.	10-11 oz-eq.
Meat & Beans	4 oz-eq.	5 oz-eq.	5-5.5 oz-eq.	5.5-6.5 oz-eq.	6.5-7 oz-eq.	7-7.5 oz-eq.	7-7.5 oz-eq.	7.5-8 oz-eq.
Milk	2-3 c.	3 c.	3 c.	3 c.	3 c.	3 c.	3 c.	3 c.
Healthy Oils	4 tsp.	5 tsp.	5 tsp.	6 tsp.	6 tsp.	7 tsp.	8 tsp.	8 tsp.

Day/Date:

Breakfast: _____ Lunch: _____

Dinner: _____ Snack: _____

Group	Fruits	Vegetables	Grains	Meat & Beans	Milk	Oils
Goal Amount						
Estimate Your Total						
Increase ⇧ or Decrease? ⇩						

Physical Activity: _____ Spiritual Activity: _____

Steps/Miles/Minutes: _____

Day/Date:

Breakfast: _____ Lunch: _____

Dinner: _____ Snack: _____

Group	Fruits	Vegetables	Grains	Meat & Beans	Milk	Oils
Goal Amount						
Estimate Your Total						
Increase ⇧ or Decrease? ⇩						

Physical Activity: _____ Spiritual Activity: _____

Steps/Miles/Minutes: _____

Day/Date:

Breakfast: _____ Lunch: _____

Dinner: _____ Snack: _____

Group	Fruits	Vegetables	Grains	Meat & Beans	Milk	Oils
Goal Amount						
Estimate Your Total						
Increase ⇧ or Decrease? ⇩						

Physical Activity: _____ Spiritual Activity: _____

Steps/Miles/Minutes: _____

Day/Date: ___

Breakfast: _____ Lunch: _____

Dinner: _____ Snack: _____

Group	Fruits	Vegetables	Grains	Meat & Beans	Milk	Oils
Goal Amount						
Estimate Your Total						
Increase ⇧ or Decrease? ⇩						

Physical Activity: _____ Spiritual Activity: _____

Steps/Miles/Minutes: _____

Day/Date: ___

Breakfast: _____ Lunch: _____

Dinner: _____ Snack: _____

Group	Fruits	Vegetables	Grains	Meat & Beans	Milk	Oils
Goal Amount						
Estimate Your Total						
Increase ⇧ or Decrease? ⇩						

Physical Activity: _____ Spiritual Activity: _____

Steps/Miles/Minutes: _____

Day/Date: ___

Breakfast: _____ Lunch: _____

Dinner: _____ Snack: _____

Group	Fruits	Vegetables	Grains	Meat & Beans	Milk	Oils
Goal Amount						
Estimate Your Total						
Increase ⇧ or Decrease? ⇩						

Physical Activity: _____ Spiritual Activity: _____

Steps/Miles/Minutes: _____

Day/Date: ___

Breakfast: _____ Lunch: _____

Dinner: _____ Snack: _____

Group	Fruits	Vegetables	Grains	Meat & Beans	Milk	Oils
Goal Amount						
Estimate Your Total						
Increase ⇧ or Decrease? ⇩						

Physical Activity: _____ Spiritual Activity: _____

Steps/Miles/Minutes: _____

Copyright 2009 First Place 4 Health. Do not duplicate without permission from First Place 4 Health.

Live It Tracker

Name: _____ Loss/gain: _____ lbs.

Date: _____ Week #: ____ Calorie Range: _____ My food goal for next week: _____

Activity Level: None, < 30 min/day, 30-60 min/day, 60+ min/day   My activity goal for next week: _____

Group	Daily Calories							
	1300-1400	1500-1600	1700-1800	1900-2000	2100-2200	2300-2400	2500-2600	2700-2800
Fruits	1.5-2 c.	1.5-2 c.	1.5-2 c.	2-2.5 c.	2-2.5 c.	2.5-3.5 c.	3.5-4.5 c.	3.5-4.5 c.
Vegetables	1.5-2 c.	2-2.5 c.	2.5-3 c.	2.5-3 c.	3-3.5 c.	3.5-4.5 c.	4.5-5 c.	4.5-5 c.
Grains	5 oz-eq.	5-6 oz-eq.	6-7 oz-eq.	6-7 oz-eq.	7-8 oz-eq.	8-9 oz-eq.	9-10 oz-eq.	10-11 oz-eq.
Meat & Beans	4 oz-eq.	5 oz-eq.	5-5.5 oz-eq.	5.5-6.5 oz-eq.	6.5-7 oz-eq.	7-7.5 oz-eq.	7-7.5 oz-eq.	7.5-8 oz-eq.
Milk	2-3 c.	3 c.	3 c.	3 c.	3 c.	3 c.	3 c.	3 c.
Healthy Oils	4 tsp.	5 tsp.	5 tsp.	6 tsp.	6 tsp.	7 tsp.	8 tsp.	8 tsp.

Day/Date:

Breakfast: _____ Lunch: _____

Dinner: _____ Snack: _____

Group	Fruits	Vegetables	Grains	Meat & Beans	Milk	Oils
Goal Amount						
Estimate Your Total						
Increase ⇧ or Decrease? ⇩						

Physical Activity: _____ Spiritual Activity: _____

Steps/Miles/Minutes: _____

Day/Date:

Breakfast: _____ Lunch: _____

Dinner: _____ Snack: _____

Group	Fruits	Vegetables	Grains	Meat & Beans	Milk	Oils
Goal Amount						
Estimate Your Total						
Increase ⇧ or Decrease? ⇩						

Physical Activity: _____ Spiritual Activity: _____

Steps/Miles/Minutes: _____

Day/Date:

Breakfast: _____ Lunch: _____

Dinner: _____ Snack: _____

Group	Fruits	Vegetables	Grains	Meat & Beans	Milk	Oils
Goal Amount						
Estimate Your Total						
Increase ⇧ or Decrease? ⇩						

Physical Activity: _____ Spiritual Activity: _____

Steps/Miles/Minutes: _____

Day/Date: ___

Breakfast: _____ Lunch: _____

Dinner: _____ Snack: _____

Group	Fruits	Vegetables	Grains	Meat & Beans	Milk	Oils
Goal Amount						
Estimate Your Total						
Increase ⇧ or Decrease? ⇩						

Physical Activity: _____ Spiritual Activity: _____

Steps/Miles/Minutes: _____

Day/Date: ___

Breakfast: _____ Lunch: _____

Dinner: _____ Snack: _____

Group	Fruits	Vegetables	Grains	Meat & Beans	Milk	Oils
Goal Amount						
Estimate Your Total						
Increase ⇧ or Decrease? ⇩						

Physical Activity: _____ Spiritual Activity: _____

Steps/Miles/Minutes: _____

Day/Date: ___

Breakfast: _____ Lunch: _____

Dinner: _____ Snack: _____

Group	Fruits	Vegetables	Grains	Meat & Beans	Milk	Oils
Goal Amount						
Estimate Your Total						
Increase ⇧ or Decrease? ⇩						

Physical Activity: _____ Spiritual Activity: _____

Steps/Miles/Minutes: _____

Day/Date: ___

Breakfast: _____ Lunch: _____

Dinner: _____ Snack: _____

Group	Fruits	Vegetables	Grains	Meat & Beans	Milk	Oils
Goal Amount						
Estimate Your Total						
Increase ⇧ or Decrease? ⇩						

Physical Activity: _____ Spiritual Activity: _____

Steps/Miles/Minutes: _____

Live It Tracker

Name: _____ Loss/gain: _____ lbs.
Date: _____ Week #: ____ Calorie Range: _____ My food goal for next week: _____
Activity Level: None, < 30 min/day, 30-60 min/day, 60+ min/day My activity goal for next week: _____

Group	Daily Calories							
	1300-1400	1500-1600	1700-1800	1900-2000	2100-2200	2300-2400	2500-2600	2700-2800
Fruits	1.5-2 c.	1.5-2 c.	1.5-2 c.	2-2.5 c.	2-2.5 c.	2.5-3.5 c.	3.5-4.5 c.	3.5-4.5 c.
Vegetables	1.5-2 c.	2-2.5 c.	2.5-3 c.	2.5-3 c.	3-3.5 c.	3.5-4.5 c.	4.5-5 c.	4.5-5 c.
Grains	5 oz-eq.	5-6 oz-eq.	6-7 oz-eq.	6-7 oz-eq.	7-8 oz-eq.	8-9 oz-eq.	9-10 oz-eq.	10-11 oz-eq.
Meat & Beans	4 oz-eq.	5 oz-eq.	5-5.5 oz-eq.	5.5-6.5 oz-eq.	6.5-7 oz-eq.	7-7.5 oz-eq.	7-7.5 oz-eq.	7.5-8 oz-eq.
Milk	2-3 c.	3 c.	3 c.	3 c.	3 c.	3 c.	3 c.	3 c.
Healthy Oils	4 tsp.	5 tsp.	5 tsp.	6 tsp.	6 tsp.	7 tsp.	8 tsp.	8 tsp.

Day/Date:

Breakfast: _____ Lunch: _____
Dinner: _____ Snack: _____

Group	Fruits	Vegetables	Grains	Meat & Beans	Milk	Oils
Goal Amount						
Estimate Your Total						
Increase ⇧ or Decrease? ⇩						

Physical Activity: _____ Spiritual Activity: _____
Steps/Miles/Minutes: _____

Day/Date:

Breakfast: _____ Lunch: _____
Dinner: _____ Snack: _____

Group	Fruits	Vegetables	Grains	Meat & Beans	Milk	Oils
Goal Amount						
Estimate Your Total						
Increase ⇧ or Decrease? ⇩						

Physical Activity: _____ Spiritual Activity: _____
Steps/Miles/Minutes: _____

Day/Date:

Breakfast: _____ Lunch: _____
Dinner: _____ Snack: _____

Group	Fruits	Vegetables	Grains	Meat & Beans	Milk	Oils
Goal Amount						
Estimate Your Total						
Increase ⇧ or Decrease? ⇩						

Physical Activity: _____ Spiritual Activity: _____
Steps/Miles/Minutes: _____

Copyright 2009 First Place 4 Health. Do not duplicate without permission from First Place 4 Health.

Day/Date: _____

Breakfast: _____   Lunch: _____

Dinner: _____   Snack: _____

Group	Fruits	Vegetables	Grains	Meat & Beans	Milk	Oils
Goal Amount						
Estimate Your Total						
Increase ⇧ or Decrease? ⇩						

Physical Activity: _____   Spiritual Activity: _____

Steps/Miles/Minutes: _____

Day/Date: _____

Breakfast: _____   Lunch: _____

Dinner: _____   Snack: _____

Group	Fruits	Vegetables	Grains	Meat & Beans	Milk	Oils
Goal Amount						
Estimate Your Total						
Increase ⇧ or Decrease? ⇩						

Physical Activity: _____   Spiritual Activity: _____

Steps/Miles/Minutes: _____

Day/Date: _____

Breakfast: _____   Lunch: _____

Dinner: _____   Snack: _____

Group	Fruits	Vegetables	Grains	Meat & Beans	Milk	Oils
Goal Amount						
Estimate Your Total						
Increase ⇧ or Decrease? ⇩						

Physical Activity: _____   Spiritual Activity: _____

Steps/Miles/Minutes: _____

Day/Date: _____

Breakfast: _____   Lunch: _____

Dinner: _____   Snack: _____

Group	Fruits	Vegetables	Grains	Meat & Beans	Milk	Oils
Goal Amount						
Estimate Your Total						
Increase ⇧ or Decrease? ⇩						

Physical Activity: _____   Spiritual Activity: _____

Steps/Miles/Minutes: _____

Copyright 2009 First Place 4 Health. Do not duplicate without permission from First Place 4 Health.

Made in the USA
Columbia, SC
18 October 2022